PSEUDOHYPACUSIS

False and Exaggerated Hearing Loss

PSEUDOHYPACUSIS

False and Exaggerated Hearing Loss

JAMES E. PECK, PhD

Associate Professor Emeritus
Otolaryngology and Communicative Sciences and Disorders
University of Mississippi Medical Center

PLURAL PUBLISHING
INC.
SAN DIEGO
OXFORD
BRISBANE

PLURAL PUBLISHING INC.

5521 Ruffin Road
San Diego, CA 92123

e-mail: info@pluralpublishing.com
Web site: http://www.pluralpublishing.com

49 Bath Street
Abingdon, Oxfordshire OX14 1EA
United Kingdom

Typeset in 11/14 Garamond Book by Flanagan's Publishing Services, Inc.
Printed in the United States of America by McNaughton and Gunn

Library of Congress Cataloging-in-Publication Data

Peck, James E., 1940-
Pseudohypacusis : false and exaggerated hearing loss / James E. Peck.
p. ; cm.
False and exaggerated hearing loss
Includes bibliographical references and index.
ISBN-13: 978-1-59756-397-0 (alk. paper)
ISBN-10: 1-59756-397-8 (alk. paper)
1. Hearing disorders—Diagnosis. 2. Audiometry. 3. Deafness—Psychological aspects. I. Title. II. Title: False and exaggerated hearing loss.
[DNLM: 1. Hearing Loss, Functional—diagnosis. 2. Hearing Loss, Functional—psychology. WV 270]
RF294.P43 2011
617.8'075—dc22

2011001756

Contents

Foreword

Since books on the subject of audiology began to be published in the 1950s, most have contained a chapter on the subject of false and exaggerated hearing loss. Because of the space limitations imposed by writing a single chapter, authors, including this writer, necessarily limited the coverage of this vast subject. This is the first time that an entire book has been devoted to this topic, resulting in all of its aspects being covered exhaustively as never before.

Although inaccurate claims of disability have been recognized for many years as a problem for clinicians and adjudicators, the dilemma leapt into prominence at the close of World War II when many U.S. service members returned to civilian life with a variety of disorders that were associated with their military service. Previously, the Veterans Administration (VA) had been a relatively small government agency, which then faced a huge problem in rehabilitation and compensation for a variety of disabilities, the largest number of which was, and continues to be, hearing loss.

The aims of VA audiology have always been twofold, to provide the maximum amount of auditory rehabilitation and to provide compensation if the hearing loss is deemed to be service connected. Proper recompense requires accurate assessment of true hearing loss. Audiologists working in the civilian area and in the military have those responsibilities in common, regardless of patient cooperation during interviewing and testing.

It is always easier and more pleasant to work with patients who are cooperative but the lack of cooperation, whether deliberate or not, does not mitigate our responsibility to diagnose and provide maximum rehabilitation. It also does not lessen the respect with which all patients must be treated. This book suggests a change in the usual concept of the person most likely to present FEHL. The traditional image has been an adult male faker. The fuller picture indicates that the person is more likely to be a child female nonfaker.

Despite many attempts by researchers, it remains extremely difficult to assess the emotional, financial, and other motivations that result in feigned or exaggerated hearing loss. Individuals often cannot understand their own psychological reasons for particular behaviors. Additionally, accurate voluntary audiometric results surely cannot be expected from those whose motivations may be considered "dishonest." So, in the final analysis, these important contributory factors are left to conjecture. However, this does not lessen the responsibility of the audiologist to determine the true hearing status of all patients regardless of their levels of active cooperation. That said, patient management becomes the primary issue. All of these factors are addressed in appropriate detail in this book.

In *Pseudohypacusis: False and Exaggerated Hearing Loss*, Dr. Peck has amassed information on the subject of this condition in ways never before accomplished. He has included all related subjects and has treated the different theories and beliefs in impartial and logical ways. This is both a practical text with adequate "how to" application and a scholarly piece. Each subject is carefully examined and exhaustively covered in unbiased ways with clear and direct writing. There is no other book, to my knowledge, with this scope and depth. It belongs on the reading lists of courses taken by candidates for the Doctor of Audiology degree and on the shelves of practicing clinicians.

Frederick N. Martin, PhD
Lillie Hage Jamail Centennial Professor Emeritus
Communication Sciences and Disorders
The University of Texas at Austin

Preface

One sees what one looks for.
One looks for what one knows.

—Anonymous

With the many dozens of books on audiology, no aspect of the field has been neglected except one: pseudohypacusis. Pseudohypacusis, or false and exaggerated hearing loss, is its own entity: it has its own literature, clinical presentation, diagnostic approach, significance, and management. Yet, even though it is one of the oldest areas in audiology, there are no books about it. This book is intended to fill that void by providing a single, comprehensive source of information covering all aspects from interview to management of this fascinating, often confusing, and frequently exasperating phenomenon.

False and exaggerated hearing loss (FEHL) does not command the interest that it used to. Writings on the topic declined in the 1980s. There also seems to be less clinical training and education on the subject now than a few decades ago. But there is no reason to suppose that the incidence of FEHL has changed. Perhaps, the subject has been crowded out by so much that is new in audiology: infant hearing loss detection programs, advanced diagnostic procedures, sophisticated hearing aid technology, cochlear implants, and so forth. Also, audiology, like all fields of endeavor—and despite our beliefs to the contrary—tends to follow fads: whatever is the latest, the most prestigious, or the most likely to get published or grant-supported. However, false hearing loss was an issue from the emergence of audiology some 70 years ago and will still be an issue 70 years from now. As time goes by, much in our current diagnostic practices and hearing aid instrumentation will become outdated because of advances in technology, biology, and medicine. But false or exaggerated hearing loss is a peculiarly human condition. It has, undoubtedly, been around as long as human nature and the experience that having a fictitious symptom—consciously or unconsciously—can have its benefits. This will always be true.

A major concept in this book is that FEHL is not always, or even usually, a simple matter of faking, but rather an indication of a psychosocial disorder. Too often, clinicians equate false hearing loss with malingering and, therefore, worthy of contempt. By definition, FEHL is not an auditory problem. But because people with FEHL come to us audiologists, and because a good many of them may well have some problem in life, it is most certainly an audiologic issue. Although reliable prevalence statistics are hard to come by, FEHL probably is more common than supposed. Indeed, in all likelihood, it is more common among children than adults. It surely must be far more common than, say, eighth cranial nerve tumors. Yet, false hearing loss is the least understood area of audiology and one that audiologists are least adept at handling in its entirety. In short, FEHL is underdetected, underappreciated, and undermanaged.

None of this is to say that people—adults or children—never feign a hearing loss for some external gain. Nor, is it implied that all persons with FEHL have a psychosocial problem. However, the literature is replete with warnings of the risk of a psychosocial difficulty. Despite abundant warnings, there is in effect no information in the literature about how to check for such risks, how to discuss and explain them, or how to approach making a referral for further management. Even outstanding books on counseling and interviewing in communicative disorders do not mention false or exaggerated hearing loss.

Audiologists can play a role, not only in uncovering a FEHL and determining genuine hearing status, but also in identifying the risk of a psychosocial disorder and directing individuals for help for any underlying problems. It is hoped that this book will give clinicians the perspective and information to do both.

This book was spurred on by a career-long interest in false and exaggerated hearing loss and the conviction that such losses often are a sign of distress. My purpose in writing it is to bring about a fuller view of false and exaggerated hearing loss and one that is more complex than commonly believed.

Acknowledgments

One of the unexpected delights in writing this book was the generous assistance from several people, some of whom were strangers.

Sally Austen, Consultant Clinical Psychologist, National Deaf Mental Health Services, Birmingham, Chair of the British Society of Mental Health and Deafness, and Honorary Lecturer, University of Northumbria, UK, gave so willingly of time and talent as a reader-editor and also as an indispensable consultant regarding psychology.

Elizabeth de Koker, PhD, private practice, Krugersdorp, Gauteng, South Africa, was an early and enthusiastic supporter of mine and whose dissertation on ASSR in pseudohypacusis is a model of thoroughness.

James W. Hall III, PhD was kind to offer to write the chapter on objective auditory measures. As if Jay did not have enough to occupy him with all his writing and global lecturing, he provided the structure and content for that chapter.

Teri A. Hamill, PhD, Professor, Audiology Department, Nova Southeastern University, Fort Lauderdale, Florida, suggested inclusion of worthwhile material and provided the sources.

Frederick N. Martin, PhD, Lillie Hage Jamail Centennial Professor Emeritus, Communication Sciences and Disorders, The University of Texas at Austin, the leading light on false hearing loss, bolstered me and made valuable suggestions throughout the four years of writing this book.

William D. Mustain, PhD, Associate Professor and Director of the Vestibular Laboratory, University of Mississippi Medical Center,

Jackson, an admired colleague and friend, served as an excellent resource regarding technology. Moreover, Bill has a keen eye for writing and improved the manuscript substantially.

Donald B. Penzien, PhD, Professor of Psychiatry and Director of Head Pain Center, Department of Psychiatry and Human Behavior, University of Mississippi Medical Center, helped significantly in getting the book underway and with matters of behavioral psychology.

The staff of the Rowland Medical Library, University of Mississippi Medical Center, was always available, obliging, and capable in assisting my research.

Gabrielle Saunders, PhD, National Center for Rehabilitative Auditory Research at the Portland, Oregon V.A. Medical Center was helpful with wording and resources about obscure auditory disorder.

Thomas Thunder, AuD, audiologist and an acoustical specialist, Acoustic Associates, Ltd., Palatine, Illinois had the major role in writing Chapter 8 on legal and forensic aspects. **William D. Domico, PhD, JD**, former audiologist and now attorney in Memphis, Tennessee, ensured the accuracy of the legal information. I had felt that this book would not be complete without a chapter on legal and forensic matters, but I was hardly qualified. Good fortune brought these two fine professionals to my attention.

Robert G. Turner, PhD, Professor, Department of Communication Disorders, Louisiana State University Health Sciences Center, New Orleans, lent me his considerable expertise on test efficiency and made fine suggestions about my wording.

Contributors

William D. Domico, PhD, JD
Domico Kyle, PLLC
Memphis, Tennessee
Chapter 9. Legal-Forensic Aspects

James W. Hall III, PhD
Clinical Professor
Department of Speech, Language, and Hearing Sciences
College of Public Health and Health Professions
University of Florida
Gainesville, Florida
Chapter 8. Objective Measures of Auditory Function

Thomas Thunder, AuD, INCE
Institute of Noise Control Engineering (Board Certified)
Acoustic Associates, Ltd.
Palatine, Illinois
Northern Illinois University
DeKalb, Illinois
Chapter 9. Legal-Forensic Aspects

To begin, I dedicate this book to three superb audiologists. The first two are my audiology fathers, Drs. Noel D. Matkin and Mark Ross. It was my great fortune to have these two fine gentlemen as professors at my master's degree program at the University of Connecticut in the 1960s during what some veteran audiologists call the "golden age" of audiology. They also became my good friends. The third audiologist is Dr Frederick N. Martin, a kind, positive friend. What models!

Also to my loving and supportive wife Pat, my patient encourager and truly best friend.

Finally, to the patients with false or exaggerated hearing loss and their families whom it was an honor to serve and who taught me so much and made my career so rewarding.

Chapter 1

TERMINOLOGY

A person who only fakes on a test is not the same as one who acts out the life of a deaf or hearing-impaired person.

—Noble, 1987, p. 2

Introduction

A person may produce invalid auditory test results for a number of reasons. However, not all such situations are considered pseudohypacusis or false or exaggerated hearing loss (FEHL). Reasons for inaccurate results include: (1) mental and motor limitations (e.g., not able to understand the procedure, unable to perform the task, or attention difficulty), (2) physical discomfort, pain, or nausea; (3) physical condition: fatigued, weak, sleepy; (4) psychological status: distraught, depressed; (5) low motivation; (6) medications affecting mental and physical status; and (7) tinnitus. Audiologists obtaining invalid results in these circumstances do not consider such findings FEHL Implicit in FEHL and kindred terms is the notion that the person is able to perform the task at hand. If not, tests results are described as invalid, and the patient may be classified as "could not test." If a patient is reasonably capable but the test performance is invalid, such results are classified as FEHL (or some related term).

Virtually every article or book chapter on false hearing loss begins by defining terms. Unlike nearly all other areas in communicative disorders, false hearing loss has many terms and words to label it. There is no confusion about or multiplicity of terms for language disorder, aphonia, conductive hearing loss, and so on. Moreover, if someone read every rationale for preferring one term over all the others, one would come away entirely bewildered. Each of three main terms—nonorganic, functional, and pseudohypacusis—has been advocated and defended as the best one. Also, the term malingering is still used, even though it has been roundly criticized by most writers on the subject. Perhaps the inevitable definitions at the outset of most any writing shows the persistent ambiguity and incomplete understanding of the nature of false hearing loss. Furthermore, the multiplicity of terms might mean that there is not simply one homogenous group of people with false or exaggerated hearing loss (see Aplin & Rowson, 1990; Austen & Lynch, 2004).

Because so many terms are used in regard to false hearing loss, confusion and misunderstanding necessarily abound. A partial list includes conversion, dissimulation, dissociative, factitious, faking, feigning, functional, hysterical, malingering, nonorganic, psychogenic, pseudohypacusis, and simulated. Selecting an appropriate designation is not a trifling exercise in semantics because proper interaction with patients and meeting their needs hinge on a correct understanding of their situation. There is great merit in using the right words in the right way.

There is another reason why it is beneficial, indeed, necessary, to sort out the more common terms used for this topic. It is a time-honored truism in psychology that how we label things influences how we think about them, and how we think about things influences how we label them. Prominent examples are words used to refer to various ethnic groups.

Considering all the above, it is necessary at the outset of this book to examine the words and phrases used with regard to false and exaggerated hearing loss.

Sorting Through the Classic Definitions

Nonorganic

A nonorganic disorder is one with no primary structural or physiologic abnormality of the organ in question. Hence, nonorganic hearing loss means apparent hearing deficit in the absence of anatomic and/or physiologic explanation (Mendel, Danhauer, & Singh, 1999; Stach, 1997).

Functional

In general medical usage, functional is synonymous with nonorganic (i.e., a disorder of function with no known organic basis per *Dorland's Illustrated Medical Dictionary*, 2003). A prime example is irritable bowel syndrome, in which there is no primary disorder of the gastrointestinal system. Thus, a functional hearing loss is one with no physiologic basis (Mendel, Danhauer, & Singh, 1999). In practice, audiologists define nonorganic or functional hearing loss operationally, namely, unexplained discrepancies among behaviors and audiometric tests with no medical evidence of an organic condition, a meaning very close to that of Ventry and Chaiklin's (1962, 1965c): "Functional hearing loss may be defined operationally as the presence of intra- or intertest discrepancies in audiometric results that are not explained by medical conditions known to be the cause of audiometric discrepancies" (Ventry & Chaiklin, 1965c, p. 179). They advocated "functional" because nonorganic does not allow for the possibility that there is some undetected, genuine organic factor.

In a different usage, functional means function that is abnormal but not pathological. For example, a "functional heart murmur" refers to a genuinely atypical valve function that is harmless and usually called innocent (Caceres & Perry, 1967; Tilkian & Conover, 2001). But probably the most powerful illustration of words having multiple meanings is using functional, ironically, to mean organic. "For [our] purposes . . . , functional hearing loss *means organic hearing loss*, that is, true pathology" (present author's emphasis) (Kesser & Friedman, 2002, p. 33).

Note that, as generally used, the terms nonorganic and functional do not mean the absence of any physical problem whatsoever. Yet, when audiologists use these terms, they mean exactly that, namely, that there is no hearing problem at all (excepting a coexisting organic hearing loss). To wit, "the loss either does not exist at all or does not exist to the degree that is indicated" (Roeser, Buckley, & Stickney, 2000, p. 237). Some have recognized this conflict and advised using "problem" instead of "loss" (e.g., Dixon & Newby, 1959). The issue is not solved by substituting one word denoting deficiency for another. Thus, it is illogical to say that a hearing loss is nonorganic or functional, when the "essential quality is precisely that it is *not* a hearing loss" (Noble, 1978, p. 228). Describing someone as having an "exaggerated hearing loss might be construed as an actual impairment of hearing even though this is not the intended case" (Engelberg, 1970, p. xiii). Hence, the terms nonorganic hearing loss and functional hearing loss are inherently self-contradictory because they describe a loss that does not exist.

Malingering

Malingering is a highly specific term meaning intentional production of false or exaggerated symptoms for external gain, such as, getting money or avoiding undesired activity (American Psychiatric Association, 2000). No audiologic test can determine what is in the patient's mind. Thus, it should never be used as a synonym for pseudohypacusis.

Psychogenic

Psychogenesis refers to production or causation of a symptom or illness by mental or psychic factors as opposed to organic ones (Shahrokh & Hales, 2003). Today, the word usually implies a conversion disorder in which psychological stresses are manifested as (converted into) symptoms, such as decreased hearing (American Psychiatric Association, 2000). A conversion disorder may be considered the converse of malingering in that there is no conscious intention to deceive, and the need is internal rather than external. The word psychogenic by its nature—meaning originating in the mind—is fundamentally vague because all our thoughts and feelings originate in the mind. "Psychogenic" is no longer used in the major psychiatric manuals of disorders, the *Diagnostic and Statistical Manual of Mental Disorders*, Fourth Edition, Text Revision, 2000 (DSM-IV TR) (American Psychiatric Association, 2000) and the *International Statistical Classification of Diseases and Related Health Problems*, 10th Revision (ICD-10) (World Health Organization, 2001).

Pseudohypacusis

The term pseudohypacusis concocted from Greek means "false hearing loss." The term made its first appearance as pseudo neural hypacusis (Brockman & Hoversten, 1960) followed by "pseudohypoacusis" (Carhart, 1961),[1] later shortened to its present form of

[1]Ironically, Carhart used this word in describing his course on tests for malingering given at a conference.

pseudohypacusis. It has come to signify invalid hearing test results, as when persons "respond to stimuli only at levels well above their true organic thresholds" but without "implying an underlying causal factor" (Olsen, 1991, p. 40). Even though many authors favor the term, "pseudohypacusis" has not gained complete acceptance in clinical parlance, possibly because it is so polysyllabic. Perhaps the best label is simply the plain English "false hearing loss," FHL, or in the case of some degree of organic impairment, "exaggerated hearing loss," EHL.[2] To cover both eventualities, a more comprehensive term would be false and exaggerated hearing loss.

In summary, the first two terms, nonorganic and functional, say that there is presentation of hearing loss but there really is no hearing loss. The next two, malingering and psychogenic, purport to say how and why a false hearing loss is presented: intentionally versus unintentionally and whether the goal is external versus internal, even though no audiologic test can determine those issues. The last, pseudohypacusis, says the hearing loss presented does not exist, or not to the extent presented, and makes no implication as to the basis for the presented hearing loss. It is the most reasonable designation. However, this writer prefers the simpler "false or exaggerated hearing loss" or its abbreviation FEHL.

Additional Problems with Terms

Preempting Elevated Thresholds by Clinical Skill

An astute clinician, who has suspicions from the outset, might choose not to plot dubious thresholds for a given patient. Instead, the clinician might keep intensity low, say 10 to 20 dB HL, and screen across several frequencies. The patient might begin to respond,

---

[2]Snyder (2001) uses "exaggerated hearing loss (EHL)" to cover all false hearing loss, even when there is no impairment at all. Because he is writing about medicolegal cases, he allows the presumption that there is likely a coexisting genuine hearing loss. Engelberg (1970) uses the phrase "exaggerated hearing level" to encompass any nonexistent impairment.

which the clinician reinforces, eventually leading to an unambiguous pass in each ear. As a result, a false hearing loss never has the chance to materialize audiometrically, a highly desirable goal (also treated later). Thus, just the claim or report of a hearing loss may qualify as a false hearing loss, even though no "hearing loss" is plotted on an audiogram. Hence, in addition to discrepancies and inconsistencies, one definition of pseudohypacusis includes merely an "alleged loss of hearing sensitivity" but no loss is found (Campbell, Peck, & Lee, 2008). This may strike some as insufficient, but that may reflect the peculiar nature of this phenomenon. FEHL is not just tone and speech thresholds on a results form.

"Faking" and "Feigning"

Probably the most common nontechnical words audiologists use to describe a person yielding invalid test results are "faking" and "feigning." To fake and to feign are nearly synonymous. As regards health or a symptom, they mean to simulate, give false appearance, represent falsely, and pretend. Both words denote that the patient's behaviors are intentionally dishonest. Although that may be the case, no audiologic data can tell what is in a patient's mind.

The ambiguity of these two words can be shown by taking a broader perspective. Even though faking (or feigning) denotes deliberate dishonesty, not all faking is a moral evil. It could be highly adaptive, such as a prisoner of war faking (feigning) some problem to seek easier treatment by the captors (Austen & Lynch, 2004). Faking also can have a reverse meaning: hiding instead of fabricating a disorder, which can also have varied moral implications. A person could hide a vision deficiency and fake normal vision by memorizing an eye chart to enter the military in time of war. Society would not encourage it but also would not consider it immoral, but instead noble and patriotic. Or a person could hide a vision deficiency to keep a job as a commercial truck driver. Although understandable, it is morally unjustifiable because of the danger to others. In any event, "faking" and "feigning" have limited value in audiology, especially as there are better alternatives.

"No Known Organic Basis"

Common to definitions of virtually all terms regarding false hearing loss is the notion of "no known organic basis." On closer examination, this component is troublesome. In the majority of cases of sensorineural hearing loss, there is no outside, verifying evidence of an organic lesion. An example of objective verification would be imaging that disclosed a tumor on the acoustic nerve. Ventry and Chaiklin's (1962) classic definition has a subtle but overlooked qualification about no corroborative medical findings. The lack of supportive medical findings does not refer to a lesion but rather to the audiometric discrepancies: "with medical examinations that rule out apparent organic conditions that might account for the discrepancies" (Ventry & Chaiklin, 1962, p. 254).

In nearly every case of sensorineural hearing impairment, the diagnosis is based on history, physical examination, and audiometric test results. It is an inference but such a robust one that "proof" of an organic lesion is hardly needed. There may be an obvious explanation for the measured hearing loss, namely, advanced age or a history of excessive sound exposure. However, neither age nor history of noise exposure is evidence of an organic lesion. Even absence of otoacoustic emissions (OAEs) is not objective proof of a sensorineural lesion, unless there is also an objective indication of normal middle ear functioning by immittance testing. Arguably, the combination of normal middle ear measures and absent OAEs constitutes objective "proof" of a sensorineural lesion. However, such testing is usually performed, not to prove a cochlear lesion, but either to help distinguish between cochlear and neural lesions or because there is some doubt about the validity of the hearing loss. The point is, most sensorineural hearing impairments are so designated on the basis of clinical judgment. Conversely, most false hearing losses are so designated on the basis of clinical judgment. This is not necessarily improper because the role of the clinician is to make sound judgments based on knowledge, experience, observations, and the information at hand.

Another difficulty with "no known organic basis" is the matter of correct diagnosis. Ventry and Chaiklin (1962) recognized the eventuality that, after classifying a hearing loss as functional, further examination may reveal an organic condition to account for the symptoms. Silver (1996) reported information suggesting that about 20% of patients diagnosed with a conversion disorder ultimately are found to have a physical sickness that accounts for the symptoms. Hence, it may be that patients had an organic disorder, but the diagnosticians initially could not find or infer one, so there was "no known organic basis." It does not mean there wasn't one.

One more significant problem with "no known organic basis" is the state of medical science at a point in time. In medical history, some disorders once thought to be functional (in the proper sense) turned out to be organic. A disorder could have been described as having "no known organic basis," because the etiology had not yet been discovered. One example is spasmodic torticollis, a painful and debilitating disorder that causes the head to lean to one side or be pulled forward or backward. Because it can be worse during times of stress, it was considered a psychiatric disorder, until research showed that it was clearly a neurologic one (National Spasmodic Torticollis Association, 2007). Thus, the phrase "no known organic basis" may be quite literally true (i.e., there may be an organic basis, but it is unknown). In the case of most sensorineural hearing losses, truly objective outside evidence is lacking. Therefore, it is not the lack of evidence of organicity that prompts clinicians to designate a patient's hearing loss as "nonorganic," but rather the overall presentation.

Inconsistencies and Discrepancies

Significance of Inconsistencies and Discrepancies

Other widespread definitional elements of false hearing loss are "inconsistencies" and "discrepancies" during an evaluation. The literature is unanimous that they are strong indicators of false hearing loss. These two words have considerable overlap involving disagreement, incompatibility, or incongruity. A related issue is reliability, which is the degree of consistency, dependability, or repeatability.

These raise two important points. First, to a significant degree, noticing inconsistencies and discrepancies and assessing reliability are matters of judgment and experience (Coles, 2001; Ventry & Chaiklin, 1962). Second, several authors caution that many persons with FEHL may display acceptable intertest reliability (Barr, 1960), indeed, "an almost phenomenal ability to repeat test results at least during a single test session" (Snyder, 2001, p. 70). Some patients even show good reliability on repeated testing on different days by different examiners (Campanelli, 1963; Lehrer, Hirschenfang, Miller, & Radpour, 1964) or over a long period of time (Dixon & Newby, 1959). In sum, although a lack of consistency in audiologic testing is "the mainstay of diagnosis" of FEHL (Pracy et al., 1996, p. 143), the presence of consistency does not rule out FEHL.

Criteria

What constitutes inconsistencies or discrepancies? There are no universally accepted criteria for intra- and intertest discrepancies. Specifying behavioral variables would be ideal, but, in reality, difficult to do because of the subtleties of human behavior (Ventry & Chaiklin, 1962). Reaching a diagnosis of FEHL essentially is based on the clinician interpreting patient behavior, which is influenced by the clinician's personality and biases (see Sharpe, 2003, p. 157; Ventry & Chaiklin, 1962).

Auditory Processing Disorder

Often, in the literature, there is a brief, almost perfunctory, statement about considering auditory processing disorders as a possible cause of inaccurate audiometric responding. Hasbrouck (1989) found that all 22 of his patients (children to adults), who had presented a "nonorganic hearing disorder," had some significant auditory processing problems. However, he does not make a causal connection except by insinuation. It seems highly unlikely that auditory processing disorders, which typically are evinced only under adverse listening conditions, could cause difficulty during conventional pure-tone threshold audiometry or simple word recognition testing in quiet.

Consciousness and Goal

Malingering Versus Psychogenic

Since the 1960s, there have been persistent divergent opinions about consciousness and goal in FEHL. The questions were: to what extent was the patient aware of what he was doing, and was the purpose for some external or some internal goal?

In a controversial and provocative view, Goldstein (1966) contended that all pseudohypacusis was deliberate, even if the person did not know why he or she was responding invalidly. He asserted that there was no such thing as psychogenic hearing loss, that is, an unrealized, subconscious condition that caused an otherwise healthy person to have truly impaired function. Goldstein's criteria to consider a hearing loss to be psychogenic were: (1) consistently failing to respond during behavioral audiometry below a certain level, but electrophysiological audiometry elicits responses to weaker sounds, and (2) the patient's behavior in daily life conforms to the voluntary thresholds. Ultimately, the diagnosis could only be confirmed if the person later demonstrated better hearing levels in all situations after successful psychiatric or psychological treatment or spontaneous remission from the underlying disorder. As no patient had met these criteria, either according to the literature or in his experience, Goldstein deduced that such persons are consciously being deceptive. The traditional dichotomy between malingering and psychogenic hearing loss can result in the erroneous concept that a person who fakes a loss for money does not have an emotional problem. He pointed out that the great majority of people who have an opportunity to obtain money falsely do not do so. Also, information at that time suggested that malingerers had personality factors, which were aberrant. Thus, all simulated hearing losses could be considered intentional and to have a psychological origin, whether the immediate precipitating event is for external gain or for some emotional need. The patient may not even be aware of the true basis for the pretense. The one certain proof of deliberate falsifying, which Goldstein did not mention, is the patient's admission, and admission is exceedingly rare (Hopkinson, 1967; Snyder, 2001).

Hopkinson (1967) and Ventry (1968) emphatically disagreed with Goldstein's position. Hopkinson questioned his criteria, adding that the only way one can know that a person malingered is if the person owns up to it, which is very rare. It was doubtful to her that there is only one kind of pseudohypacusis, as Goldstein implied. Either way, Hopkinson contended that the audiologist's job was to evaluate hearing, not determine whether a false hearing loss was deliberate or psychogenic, even though those are interesting questions. Moreover, she challenged the idea that audiologists should or could identify whether a behavior was willful. Ventry (1968) also took issue with Goldstein's criteria by using the literal (and now outdated) meaning of psychogenic as originating in the mind; as all ideas originate in the mind, psychogenic does not distinguish between conscious and unconscious motivation. On the other hand, he made a strong case that there was such a thing as psychogenic (i.e., unconscious) hearing loss, in agreement with Hopkinson, and presented a convincing example.

Traditionally, the element of consciousness has been divided into those two categories: total as in malingering and none as in psychogenic. Many authors specifically portray consciousness in FEHL as lying along a continuum rather than just at either end (Roeser et al., 2000; Snyder, 2001). Others (e.g., Goldstein, 1966) see a discontinuity between the two types of behavior. Among all writers on the subject, Noble (1978) makes the strictest dichotomy between volitional fakery on one hand and unconscious attempts to meet a psychological need on the other. The former is malingering, which is dishonesty but not a psychiatric disorder. The latter is a conversion disorder, a psychiatric disturbance requiring mental health intervention. In Noble's view, malingering should not be included in "nonorganic hearing loss" because the individuals know full well they have no hearing loss. They fake a loss only in the clinical setting but otherwise make no pretense of being hearing impaired outside of the clinic. Persons with a conversion disorder have a true nonorganic hearing loss, per Noble, in that they believe they have a loss, and they function as though they were hearing impaired, both in and out of the test situation.

Factitious Disorder

In addition to malingering and psychogenic, there is a third category of false symptoms, factitious disorder, in which the presentation is done consciously but to meet some internal need.

> . . . Factitious Disorder is the intentional production of physical or psychological signs or symptoms, . . . fabrication of subjective complaints (e.g., pain), . . . falsification of objective signs . . . , self-inflicted conditions . . . , exaggeration or exacerbation of preexisting general medical conditions . . . , or any combination or variation of these. The motivation for the behavior is to assume the sick role. External incentives are absent. (American Psychiatric Association, 2000)

Presumably, the gains are obtaining solicitous attention, being cared for, dispensation from usual responsibilities, or even the satisfaction of fooling-manipulating the medical system (Miller, 2008).

Factitious disorder might be compatible with Goldstein's notion of patients being aware of their deception but unaware of why they do it. Indeed, perhaps the reason that so many writers consider their patients to fall somewhere in between the two extremes of malingering and conversion disorder is because many of those patients actually had a factitious disorder. Put another way, the old model was incomplete.

Austen and Lynch Model

In their landmark 2004 article, Austen and Lynch pointed out the inadequacy of the common either/or concept of FEHL, that is, malingering versus conversion disorder. They incorporated factitious disorder as a bridge between the two extremes because it contains elements of both, intentional feigning and internal needs. Accordingly, Austen and Lynch devised an innovative, illuminating, and practical model of FEHL having two dimensions, the degree of intention in producing invalid results on one axis, and the nature of the resultant gains, external versus internal, on the other axis. The diagnosis among these three categories rests on the motivation, which is a combination of the two dimensions, degree of intention and the resultant gains. Note that they use the more neutral "intent" instead of consciousness in line with current classification systems.

The Austen and Lynch model of classifying FEHL can be summarized this way

malingering:	intentional and external need
factitious:	intentional and internal need
conversion disorder:	unintentional and internal need

The concept of these three categories—malingering, factitious, and conversion—has a dual benefit. First, the categories can be applied individually for diagnostic classification. Second, they can be seen on a continuum for purposes of management. For example, at times, a conversion based hearing loss can also provide an external gain, and an external gain does not exclude meeting psychological needs. FEHLs can result from blends of thoughts and emotions. Moreover, patients may move along the two continua, or shift back and forth as to the degree of intention or the locus of need as time goes on.

Austen and Lynch (2004) contend that audiologists are ideally placed, not only to detect false hearing loss early, but also to discern cues that will aid in diagnosis and management. Thus, it is their responsibility to gain as much information as possible. They must work closely in multidisciplinary team fashion with other health care professionals, including primary care providers and those in mental health. Their purview is not to assess intent and locus of need or to surmise a diagnosis; ultimately, that clinical function lies with the mental health professional (S. Austen, personal communication, December 1, 2007).

Operational Definition of False and Exaggerated Hearing Loss

What should the focus be in defining false hearing loss, the *test results* (the inconsistencies and discrepancies), or the *patient* (the source of erroneous results)? This author thinks a full definition should not be either/or but include both. It has to include test results, for those are part of the nature of, and key to, discovering the phenomenon. But it also has to include the patient because the patient is the source of those results.

Given all the above, we now can try to construct a practical, comprehensive, accurate definition of FEHL. The definition offered is operational yet recognizes the prime role of clinical judgment. It specifies both test outcome (invalid) and patient behaviors (inconsistencies within and beyond audiologic testing). In reality, false hearing loss is a diagnostic impression based on a constellation of considerations, often more a collection of uncertainties rather than solid data, such as, atypical nontest behaviors, test discrepancies, lack of a plausible history, no supportive medical findings, in short, the clinical picture "not making sense." To put it in rather colloquial but pithy terms, experienced clinicians have the feeling of, "I know it when I see it."

The critical elements of the definition are: (1) presenting hearing loss that does not exist or not to the degree presented, (2) in that test results are judged invalid, (3) in view of inconsistent responses, or (4) discrepancies between and among tests and with nontest behaviors, (5) without a logical history or medical findings that explain such test results, (6) while making no implication about psychological factors.

Our definition, then, is:

> FEHL is an apparent hearing loss that does not exist, or not to the degree presented, as manifested by unexplained test inconsistencies and discrepancies, but without implication about psychological factors.

With the problem framed about as well as can be hoped for, we are ready to look at this phenomenon in greater breadth and depth, beginning with its emergence in audiology decades ago and the early tools that were used for its assessment.

Chapter 2

HISTORICAL PERSPECTIVE

Electrophysiologic testing has generally been done because behavioral inconsistencies led the audiologist to suspect better auditory sensitivity than could be estimated from behavioral audiometry.

—Goldstein, 1966, p. 345

Introduction

Reports on false hearing loss extend back more than a hundred years (see Berk & Feldman, 1958), but the information is sparse. In what must be one of the earliest writings, Heller in 1894 applied the expression "psychic deafness" to "functional" hearing loss to distinguish it from organic hearing loss (see Broad, 1980). Most of the early articles on adults explicitly or implicitly dealt with compensation, and those on children dealt with psychological problems, a dichotomy that probably is still accurate today.

The mid-20th century saw a dramatic increase in professional attention paid to hearing impairment for two reasons: World War II with its massive numbers of people with damaged hearing and the availability of civilian and military compensation. During that time, several tests were devised to identify FEHL and to determine genuine hearing sensitivity. Although most were fairly effective, they were somewhat intricate and time-consuming or required specialty equipment. With time, they were superseded by better procedures. Even so, the procedures of that era are educational about human hearing. Also, because of the considerable attention given FEHL, probably many more clinicians of that era were attuned to false hearing loss than clinicians since the 1980s. Now, much from that bygone period has mostly historical value but value, nonetheless. This chapter gives a historical view of that epoch.

Compensation and Disability

A prime cause—if not the prime cause—of FEHL among adults has been the opportunity to obtain money through compensation (Coles, 2001). The two major sources of compensation are industry and the military. In industry, it is based on workers' compensation (originally workmen's compensation), a program of business insurance, required by law, that provides payments for work-related injuries, illnesses, or disabilities, and for medical expenses and rehabilitation without regard to a finding of negligence of either party. Prior to compensation laws, workers had to go through long, expensive legal action under common law and even then with the possibility of not recovering damages.

Compensation laws were first adopted in Germany in 1884, in Britain in the 1890s, and in the United States in the early 1900s. The two driving forces were the industrial age with its great increase in the number of injuries, and workers' agitations to obtain the right of injured workers to compensation. The purpose was to compensate workers for time when they were unable to work and, therefore, unable to earn. Wage replacement was, and is, usually a percentage of the actual wage, generally, one-half to two-thirds of an injured worker's lost income. The thinking was that accidents were inevitable, and compensating workers was a reasonable cost of business.

The American Employee's Compensation Act of 1908 allowed compensation for loss of earnings from, among other things, traumatic sudden deafness caused by an accident (Noble, 1978). In the 1920s and 1930s, U.S. laws began to expand beyond accidental injury to cover diseases arising out of the employment environment, including the cumulative effects of job conditions. Furthermore, the laws no longer required a demonstrable loss of wages. By mid-century, compensation legislation covered any occupationally related disease.

Workers' compensation laws differ significantly from other personal injury laws. They were not intended to be punitive to the employer. As noted above, negligence on the part of the employer or the employee generally is irrelevant to determining compensability. However, for some situations, the employee might have the burden of proving that a condition was caused entirely or in part by the employment (Gale Group, 1998). For example, a company may require expert opinion on whether a hearing loss was due solely to the worker's job and not also due to activities outside the workplace. Consequently, what was intended to provide the employer and employee with a harmonious and benevolent resolution of a work injury often results in contentious disputes and costly litigation (Gale Group, 1998).

Although designed to protect the worker from economic distress or ruin, workers' compensation law also benefited the employer. It conferred some protection on companies from being sued for workplace conditions that caused injury or illness. In other words, it was a matter of economics as well as one of humanitarian concern for the quality of life of a person with permanent injuries (Noble, 1978). Another side effect was that the additional business expense of compensation insurance was passed on to consumers. Indeed, workers' compensation has been criticized as an expensive component of doing business, one made more so by undetected fraud.

There were two additional consequences of workers' compensation. A positive one was improved working conditions. Companies had an economic incentive to create safer working sites and institute programs to minimize the number of claims and, in turn, reduce their premiums. An unfavorable outcome was giving workers an incentive to feign or exaggerate injuries to receive wage loss benefits (see Gale Group, 1998; Siegel & Shim, 2005). With the favorable legal environment by the late 1940s and 1950s, there was a surge in compensation claims (Noble, 1978).

In addition to World War II and legally mandated compensation in employment, there was a coming together of several other factors that increased the attention given to claims of hearing impairment: rapidly growing industrialization worldwide, decades of legal precedence for compensation, better testing and greater awareness of hearing loss, and recognition of the humanitarian need for just recompense for an impairment in performing activities of daily living. As the opportunity grew for monetary gain, undoubtedly so did the frequency of dishonest claims of illness and disability. Further fuel was the model that a greater abnormality merited a greater compensation, which seems logical and fair. Nonetheless, it is equally logical that such a paradigm encouraged people to present a false symptom or magnify a real one. With regard to hearing, the issue can be framed as "dollars for decibels," which would entice a person to present, as much as possible, a nonexistent hearing loss or exaggerate the degree of a true loss, whether related to military service, workplace, or personal injury.

The financial implications must be enormous, given the prevalence of workplace injuries, including noise-induced hearing loss (De Koker, 2004). Matters are made worse by paying undeserved compensation. Also, attempts to falsify or exaggerate hearing loss result in the additional expense of reevaluations and lost productivity by having workers away their jobs. Of the many millions of dollars paid by the Veterans Administration for service-connected disabilities annually, a sizable portion is related to hearing impairment (Martin, 2009). How many veterans have received money for false or exaggerated hearing loss cannot be known, because the VA does not keep statistics on FEHL among military veterans (Rintelmann & Schwan, 1999).

Prevalence in the 1940s and 1950s

How common a problem is can be expressed in two ways, prevalence and incidence. These terms are similar but not synonymous. Prevalence is the number of cases of a disease or disorder existing at a given time. Incidence is the number of new cases of a disease or disorder occurring in a given time span, typically, a year. Simplistically put, they address the questions, "How many total cases?" versus "How many new cases?"

There are few trustworthy data, regardless of era, on either the prevalence or incidence of false or exaggerated hearing loss. There are so many factors that can enter into the picture. To begin with, there are no standard criteria for what constitutes FEHL; rather, there are vague behavioral indicators, such as inconsistent responding, which are highly subject to clinical acumen and judgment. Also, as mentioned in the Chapter 1, many false responders can be quite consistent during audiometric testing.

Many false hearing losses, especially in adults, are overlaid on organic impairments and, thus, more likely to be missed. Practice patterns can influence the statistics. For example, some clinicians are more likely to screen for evoked otoacoustic emissions on a routine basis and, therefore, presumably are more likely to discover an invalid result. Another matter in the calculus is the duration of a condition, short- versus long-term. Not every patient who presents FEHL continues to do so for long durations; indeed some relinquish the "loss" during one session or by the next visit. Finally, any count of cases can include only the ones that are detected. Undoubtedly, some slip through. Hence, true prevalence is unknowable.

The biggest problem by far in obtaining valid prevalence estimates is the population reported on, which is associated with test site. Settings that see large numbers of people regarding compensation report rates of FEHL that are an order of magnitude greater than those seen in general otolaryngology and audiology practices. In sum, one is left with clinical impressions, sketchy articles, and reports on highly disparate groups.

The preponderance of literature in the postwar period concerned active and veteran military personnel and, therefore, adults. Rather than give data, most early writers made general statements or reported a sense that FEHL increased among military personnel after World War II, certainly a reasonable probability. Gleason (1958) cited reports from 1946 to 1956 showing that rates of FEHL varied from 8 to 35% in military audiology centers. In Gleason's own study, 30% of the referrals to the army hospital were inconsistent responders. Johnson, Work, and McCoy (1956) reported that the number of false service-connected hearing losses rose impressively from about 12% to almost 50% in the decade following World War II.

Historical and Obsolete Tests

One of the oldest tests for FEHL is the Stenger test, yet it is hardly obsolete. (The Stenger test is treated in detail in Chapter 7, Special Behavioral Tests.) As early as 1923, Czubak (1923) praised the Stenger test as easy and infallible for detecting "simulated" total hearing loss in one ear (and decried that it received no attention).

In 1928, Guttman described a "new method" to identify malingered unilateral deafness. Tones of identical frequency were presented to both ears simultaneously. The intensity of the tone to the alleged deaf ear was raised until the patient stopped responding.

Guttman knew that, if the poor ear were truly deaf, the tone in the good ear would remain audible. He apparently was unaware that he was using the already known Stenger test (perhaps supporting Czubak's lament).

Another old test, the Lombard, is based on the Lombard effect of reflexively raising one's voice when in a loud place. The test involves presenting a masking noise to an ear or ears, while a patient reads a passage, and noticing if and at what level the patient's vocal loudness increases. A person with true hearing loss speaking when there is no noise and then when there is noise will not change vocal intensity. But a person with false hearing loss will raise the voice when noise is present to compensate for the lessened auditory self-monitoring. If voice loudness is increased when the noise is below admitted speech threshold, the threshold is in error. The Lombard test has several weaknesses. Recognizing a change in loudness is dependent on the clinician's judgment. The test does not provide reliable information on genuine threshold. Finally, a knowledgeable or insightful patient may resist the effects of loud interfering noise and maintain a consistent loudness. In the literature of the last two decades, the Lombard test has been relegated to minor historical status or is not mentioned at all.

Taylor (1949) was among the first to use an experimental approach to assess the effectiveness of tests for detecting false hearing loss. Some of his subjects had normal hearing and others had impaired hearing, but all were told to deny any hearing in one ear. He administered four tests with what he called the "fairly recently developed audiometer." All four tests generally were useful for detection and for a degree of threshold prediction.

A number of alternative approaches were devised to detect FEHL and to measure hearing sensitivity. Some of the creative attempts drew on modalities that were popular at the time. At one time the U.S. Army employed sodium pentothal ("truth serum"), when false hearing loss did not resolve through other means (Martin, 1946). Along with the light state of reduced consciousness, there was heavy use of suggestibility. Of all the cases studied, fewer than 12% were psychogenic. In cases of blast-induced hearing loss, 38% were purely psychogenic or had a large psychogenic overlay. Another modality was hypnosis, not for treatment but for diagnostic testing (Hallewell, Goetzinger, Allen, & Proud, 1966). Although hypnosis was effective in obtaining better thresholds, it was not adopted because of the lengthy session involved and the impracticality of having a hypnotist on hand. A third example of adapting what was popular at the time is conditioned response testing. In one study (Galloway & Butler, 1956), a flash of light was paired with pure-tone stimuli to condition an eyelid blink. Subjects produced conditioned eyelid responses at 5- to 10-dB Sensation Level (SL), but the procedure was impractical because it required too much time to achieve the conditioning.

Miller, Fox, and Chan (1968) suggested three modifications to pure tone testing with children: (1) telling when a descending, continuously-on tone was no longer heard, (2) judging (as a ploy) whether one tone was louder, the same or softer than another tone of a pair while gradually lowering the intensity of the tone pairs until no response, and (3) responding to signals by saying "yes" or "no." Only the "yes-no" test has remained in use and is discussed further in Chapter 6, Conventional Behavioral Audiometry.

Electrodermal Audiometry

Electrodermal audiometry (EDA) appeared in the late 1940s as an objective, electrophysiologic test of hearing to be used when voluntary responses were questionable or difficult to obtain. It used a classical conditioning paradigm of pairing an unconditioned stimulus (US) with a conditioned stimulus (CS) to establish a conditioned response (CR). In EDA, the unconditioned stimulus was a mild but unpleasant electric shock, which elicited an unconditioned response (UR) of decreased electrical skin resistance. The conditioned stimulus was a pure tone or speech. Once conditioning was established, the sound alone caused the decreased skin resistance, which was the conditioned response. The following diagram shows the process.

US → UR

US + CS → UR

CS → CR

The change in skin resistance in EDA is called the psychogalvanic skin response (PGSR). The PGSR results from a minute, momentary output from sweat glands. Sweat has chemicals that are conductors of electricity, so resistance suddenly drops. In EDA, recording electrodes were attached to the fingertips, and the shock electrodes usually were affixed to the forearm. After some presentations of the paired tone and shock, just the tone was presented and any change in skin resistance recorded. Signal level was varied until the lowest level was identified that caused a change in skin resistance. Tones were the more common signal in EDA, but speech in the form of spondaic words was an alternative signal (Hopkinson, 1978). A specific spondee was targeted as the conditioned stimulus and paired with the shock.

Although EDA was a so-called objective test in that the patient did not actively participate, a great deal of subjectivity was involved. The tester had to make judgments about acceptable response amplitude, number of responses necessary to be accepted as a genuine indication of hearing, response latency, the need to alter the reinforcement schedule, and whether extraneous movements were excessive and causing artifact.

When successful, EDA was quite reliable and valid. EDA thresholds often were shown to agree ±5 dB with voluntary pure-tone thresholds. Unfortunately, a significant proportion of patients could not be conditioned (Rintelmann & Schwan, 1999). By the early 1970s, EDA was being overtaken by evoked auditory potentials testing (Hopkinson, 1973). Also, there long had been ethical and legal questions of administering an unpleasant electric shock to humans, even though the shock was mild (Rintelmann & Schwan, 1999).

Doerfler-Stewart Test

Doerfler and Stewart (1946) recognized that some persons with FEHL could be consistent responders. They surmised that patients set up a yardstick of loudness as a criterion of when to respond. This patient strategy is effective in quiet environments, such as a hearing test room. The key to uncovering false hearing loss was disrupting a person's loudness yardstick. Therefore, Doerfler and Stewart devised a test to do just that.

Their test (sometimes called the D-S test) obtains thresholds for speech in quiet, for speech in noise, and for noise only. For persons exaggerating their thresholds, hearing different types of sound, sometimes simultaneously and sometimes separately, and at varying intensities, creates loudness confusion and, hence, inconsistency. In contrast, valid responders maintain the same speech recognition threshold (SRT). Here is an outline of the procedure (Doerfler & Stewart, 1946; Hopkinson, 1973, 1978):

1. First, an SRT is established in ascending manner: SRT_1.
2. To that is added 5 dB, called SRT_1 + 5, to ensure that the next task is fairly easy.
3. Noise is introduced at the lowest level and gradually increased until the patient no longer repeats words; this is the noise interference level (NIL).
4. The noise level is raised 20 dB to prevent hearing the speech.
5. With this loud noise on, word presentation level is lowered, soon followed by also reducing the noise level, until the patient either begins to respond again or no longer responds when noise has been reduced to 0 dB.
6. A second SRT in quiet is established: SRT_2.
7. A noise detection threshold (NDT) is found (in the original article, the noise reception threshold), the level at which the patient is first aware of the noise alone.

Those five values—SRT_1, SRT_1 +5, NIL, SRT_2, and NDT—are compared in various ways. For example, the SRTs should agree, and the NIL and the NDT should correlate fairly well.

A major drawback of the D-S test is glaringly obvious in the above outline: its complexity. Not only was performing the test arduous, but interpretation was complicated and time-consuming. Each clinic had to establish its own norms. Also, the test gave only qualitative information and not quantitative information as to genuine hearing. The D-S test was somewhat effective and some modifications helped, but the many negatives outweighed its benefits.

Delayed Auditory Feedback

When we perform a motor act that produces a sound, there is a very close correspondence between action and sound. But, if we hear the sound slightly after the act, it disrupts our auditory monitoring and alters our motor pattern. Similarly, when we speak, we hear ourselves instantaneously. If we hear our own speech slightly delayed, our speech is disrupted. The use of delayed auditory feedback (DAF) was developed in the 1950s to study sensory monitoring and was adapted as a test for FEHL by delaying feedback of one's speech.

The procedure required a tape recorder that could be in the record mode and the playback mode at the same time. The delay was the result of the physical distance between the record head and playback head and the speed of the tape going between the two heads. When people listened to themselves talk in the DAF condition, they had the unnatural experience of hearing themselves a split second after speaking, which upset their speech. A delay of about 0.18 sec. was the most effective in disrupting speech.

In the test situation, the patient read a passage while wearing earphones. Patients were not told that they would hear anything unusual during testing. First, the person read with no feedback and then read with the unexpected delayed feedback. Speech changes included slowing down, speeding up, hesitating, repeating sounds or "stuttering," talking louder, or having a vocal quaver.

Because the test was done under earphones, it could be monaural or binaural. By controlling the intensity of the feedback, the clinician could determine at what level the feedback became audible to the patient, that is, the point of speech breakdown. If the hearing loss were false, speech would be affected when the delayed feedback level was below the voluntary speech threshold. Because subjects were not expecting to hear themselves a moment after speaking, the changes in their speech were immediate and usually quite obvious.

For most who have experienced DAF, such as this author, the effect is quite powerful, dramatic, and hard to resist. That made DAF fairly effective in uncovering FEHL. But some persons could "beat the test," that is, keep up a fairly consistent reading pattern. DAF also was deficient in quantifying true hearing because, for normal hearing individuals, the sensation level (SL) to produce the effect spanned a substantial range of 20 to 40 dB. Moreover, a coexisting sensorineural disorder with recruitment lowered the SL at which DAF effects occurred. It was hazardous to infer an SRT (other than normal), because a person might happen to have an organic impairment of unknown magnitude (Rintelmann & Schwan, 1991).

DAF was improved as a hearing test by requiring the patient not to speak but in stead to tap a specified rhythmic pattern (Ruhm & Cooper, 1962). A typical pattern was (• • • • • • •). While wearing earphones, the subject tapped on a mechanical noiseless key out of sight. Tapping the key produced a nearly simultaneous brief tone. First, the tapping was done with no delay to be sure that the patient could perform the task. Some could not or would not (Martin, 2009). Then, the tone was delayed by 200 ms. Hearing the tone out of sync with the motor act disturbed the ability to maintain the same tapping pattern and pressure. Because the effect occurred at 5 dB SL, one could extrapolate genuine thresholds reasonably well (Ruhm & Cooper, 1962).

The tone DAF test had good validity. Persons with organic hearing impairments had close agreement among conventional threshold audiometry, EDA, and tone DAF (Ruhm & Cooper, 1964). In contrast, those with FEHL had good agreement only between EDA and DAF, both of which yielded better thresholds than conventional voluntary thresholds. Also, tone DAF was largely unaffected by knowledge of the test or by practice, at least at low SL (Martin & Shipp, 1982; Monro & Martin, 1977). However, the span of altered tap thresholds can be 5 to 15 dB SL and even as high as 40 dB (Alberti 1970; Martin & Shipp, 1982).

In summary, speech DAF was moderately successful, and tone DAF was even better. Tone DAF was fairly rapid, highly accurate, and permitted a reasonably good estimate of tone thresholds. But its popularity faded, as evaluation of the auditory brainstem response became widespread. With equally good or better procedures, there is not a market nowadays for a dedicated DAF system.

Békésy Audiometry

Békésy or automatic audiometry was developed so that people could plot their own thresholds across frequencies. Patients controlled intensity to trace their thresholds for both an interrupted (or pulsed) tone and for a continuous tone, as the audiometer automatically swept across the audiometric range. For persons with normal hearing, the thresholds were the same. In contrast, people with sensorineural pathologies usually had some abnormal auditory fatigue; thus, their thresholds for the continuous signal were poorer than for the interrupted signal. Different degrees of auditory fatigue resulted in different patterns—the four classic Békésy types—which were useful in distinguishing cochlear from neural hearing losses (Jerger, 1960).

In 1961, Jerger and Herer (1961) found an "unexpected dividend" from Békésy audiometry. They found three children with FEHL who produced a reverse relationship of poorer thresholds for the interrupted tone than for the continuous tone. Rintelmann and Harford (1963) encountered another nine of 10 children with FEHL who traced the same relationship. This became the Békésy Type V and was seen as a sign of false hearing loss. Apparently, the patient tries to equate the loudness of the two types of signals, and because an interrupted tone is not on all the time, it seems not as loud as a continuous tone. Rintelmann and Harford (1967) defined Type V as showing separations between continuous and interrupted tone tracings of 10 dB over a range of frequencies and at some point at least 15 dB of separation. Using these criteria, 76% of their patients who had FEHL produced a Type V pattern, and no normal listeners and only a few hearing-impaired listeners plotted a Type V.

If the loudness of an interrupted tone was less than that of a constant tone, then longer interruptions might reduce the loudness even more. In classic Békésy audiometry, the interrupted tone was on 200 ms and off 200 ms. Lengthening the off-time to 800 ms caused normal hearing subjects to trace higher intensity levels when trying to maintain the loudness of an initial loudness reference (Hattler, 1968). When the 200 and 800 ms off-time paradigms were applied to a group of patients, the lengthened off-time (LOT) resulted in a wider separation between pulsed and continuous tones in the FEHL group but not in the organic hearing-impaired group (Hattler, 1970). The sensitivity of the standard off-time test in detecting FEHL was 40%, whereas that of the lengthened off-time test was 95%.

A different Békésy variation compared tracings begun at a very low level with tracings begun at a very high level (Hood, Campbell, & Hutton, 1964). This was the Békésy ascending descending gap evaluation or BADGE. First, tracings were obtained for continuous and pulsed tones starting at the lowest level. Listeners raised the intensity until they first heard the signal and then responded (ascending condition). Next, a pulsed tone was begun 40 to 60 dB above the ascending "threshold," and subjects lowered the intensity until they no longer heard the signal and stopped responding (descending condition). Persons responding validly traced the same thresholds regardless of the initial level. In contrast, FEHL patients tended to produce a gap between the thresholds, the descending thresholds being higher than the ascending thresholds. The BADGE was about 70% efficient in separating true responders from false responders.

Chaiklin (1990) combined the ascending-descending concept with lengthened off time. He had subjects trace thresholds starting at a high level 25 dB above the poorest ascending levels. This was the descending LOT or DELOT test. It was faster to administer and easier to interpret than the standard LOT. With separations generally 10 dB wider than with the usual LOT test, 29% more in the FEHL group traced positive patterns. Sensitivity for FEHL was 100% with the DELOT versus 71% with the regular LOT test.

Standard Békésy audiometry was fairly successful in detecting FEHL. However, it offered no information about true organic hearing levels and was untrustworthy with children. In its modified forms, Békésy testing had good sensitivity, identifying 70% or more of pseudohypacusics, and a low false-positive rate of less than 5% in nonpseudohypacusics. But because Békésy audiometry was replaced by better ways to test for eighth cranial nerve tumors, which was Békésy audiometry's primary application at the time, Békésy audiometry for any purpose faded.

Audiologic and Psychosocial Characteristics

Audiologic Patterns

During the 1960s, Drs. Ira Ventry and Joseph Chaiklin were the most prolific writers on FEHL. In 1965, as audiologists with the Veterans Administration, they produced a landmark monograph on their multidisciplinary research of false and exaggerated hearing loss in veterans (Ventry & Chaiklin, 1965d). Their goals were to: (1) evaluate the efficiency of several procedures used to arrive at a diagnosis of FEHL, (2) analyze error behavior during pure-tone and speech audiometry, and (3) identify audiologic, psychological, and psychiatric variables that might distinguish between those individuals whose FEHL eventually resolves from those in whom it persists.

Their sample was 100 male veterans being seen for compensation for hearing loss. A group of 64 subjects had signs of FEHL and a comparison group of 36 subjects had no evidence of FEHL. The subjects were hospitalized for a few days to undergo extensive multispecialist evaluation. Medically, the FEHL and non-FEHL groups were indistinguishable. Forty-seven men from the FEHL group were positive on PGSR testing (the other 17 could not be conditioned). The mean invalid component in each ear for the speech frequencies was 28 dB and for speech was 18 dB. The range of the invalid components was wide, 8 to 48 dB for tones and 3 to 33 dB for speech. Of those 47 subjects positive by PGSR, 39 presented bilateral losses, both symmetrical and asymmetrical, leaving 8 who displayed a unilateral loss.

The most efficient indicator of FEHL was a discrepancy between the spondee threshold and pure-tone average (speech threshold at least 12 dB below pure tone average), which identified 70% of the subjects. Next was the 1000-Hz test-retest measure (at least a 15-dB discrepancy), which identified 66%. The two Stenger tests, tone and speech (positive meant at least 15 dB below voluntary thresholds), were the least efficient of the measures, identifying only 43% and 40% of the cases, respectively. Ventry and Chaiklin recognized that the criterion they had used of a 15-dB ear difference was too narrow. The accuracy of the Stenger tests was best when the voluntary threshold difference between the two ears was beyond 40 dB.

The two groups differed by types of spondee error. Subjects in the FEHL group gave more half-stimulus responses, more one-syllable responses not contained in the stimulus, and more no-response and total errors. After counseling the subjects about test discrepancies, the likelihood of the FEHL resolving was significantly related to the magnitude of the initial loss but not to psychological variables. An initial false component less than 35 dB was correlated with far greater probability of later resolution. Ventry and Chaiklin's findings regarding social and psychological characteristics are discussed in the following section

Psychosocial Characteristics

As has been shown, the preponderance of literature in the early years was on detection of FEHL and measurement of genuine thresholds in adults. However, some writers addressed the characteristics of persons presenting invalid audiometric results.

Several of the papers from the 1940s and 1950s dealt with the supposed symbolic significance of the ear and hearing (see Broad, 1980). Some of the literature had a distinctly Freudian psychoanalytical view of symbolism, psychodynamics, and psychosexual development, for example, the ear as an orifice that can be stimulated or penetrated. False hearing loss was interpreted as a "psychic" response to difficult environmental circumstances. A person can use hearing to maintain homeostasis by accepting pleasant (nonthreatening) acoustic stimuli and rejecting unpleasant (threatening) stimuli. Even though some of those viewpoints may be outdated, they give a remarkably different yet noteworthy look at the psychological significance of the ear and hearing. Some of the concepts, such as the role of hearing to maintain homeostasis, may continue to hold some validity.

One of the earliest systematic studies of the psychological characteristics was by Gleason in 1958. He compared 287 consecutive military patients who were deemed to be either consistent or inconsistent during audiometry. The proportion of inconsistent responders was 30%. As many as 85% among the inconsistent group had psychological problems but were not mentally ill. The psychological problems included emotional immaturity, instability, inadequate response to societal demands, and feelings of anxiety and inferiority. Gleason considered their audiometric exaggerations to be at an unconscious level. He concluded that audiologic inconsistency was part of a generalized personality disturbance.

In addition to the audiologic aspects, part of the comprehensive Ventry and Chaiklin study examined the social and psychological characteristics of their subjects at the VA facility (Trier & Levy, 1965). A typical subject in each group (FEHL and non-FEHL) had a fairly stable life. The FEHL group scored statistically lower than the non-FEHL group on some measures but not on others. For example, the FEHL group was slightly lower on measures of verbal intelligence. In addition, they had mild indications of less emotional stability and significantly more complaints of tinnitus and also of more severe tinnitus. As a group, they earned on average $2,000 less per annum than the non-FEHL group. The authors' inference was that those subjects, with their minor limitations, had less confidence to provide for themselves and their families, and being aware of the chance to get more money, they exaggerated their hearing losses. Because exaggerating a problem for gain is socially frowned upon, Trier and Levy reasoned that feeling deceitful would, in turn, lower one's self-esteem. Even though the FEHL group had a less favorable profile, the differences were small, and on some measures there were no differences.

Noble (1978) judged the Ventry-Chaiklin study to have serious flaws. The study sample was so narrow that the significance of the results and their generalizabilty were limited. Necessarily, the population was highly skewed toward: (1) male military veterans, (2) who had been in situations that often involved exposure to very strong sound, or (3) had had that exposure under the stressful experience of combat, and (4) were aware that compensation was available for permanent injuries, indeed, the greater the abnormality, the greater the recompense. Yet, even though some individuals showed signs of FEHL, many others did not. The veterans were hospitalized, in effect "imprisoned" in Noble's thinking, and coerced into a study unaware that they were subjects in a study. Even though they were no longer in the armed forces, they still were hospitalized and put through rigorous testing without informed consent. Furthermore, Noble felt that there was a sense of threat in being told it was necessary to be in a hospital for 3 to 4 days because of the test discrepancies. Out of all the evaluations, the biggest difference between the groups was that the FEHL men earned $2,000 less per year than the non-FEHL men. Nothing else appeared to account for the differences in behavior as much as the difference in economic situation and potential improvement.

Although Noble makes many useful points, the absence of similar criticisms in all the years since the Ventry-Chaiklin report suggests that there is still merit in what those investigators found. At a time when audiology was coming of age, Ventry and Chaiklin tried to bring some order to terminology and protocol, and they brought a great deal of attention to FEHL in an organized, thoughtful way.

Summary

There were a great many people with hearing impairment in the mid-20th century due to World War II and global mechanization. Concomitantly, there must have been an increase in FEHL related to psychological trauma of combat and to the availability of military and civilian compensation. Veterans were entitled to payments for service-connected injuries, and workers were eligible for compensation for all occupational injuries or illnesses on a no-fault basis. The rule was the greater the disability, the greater the compensation. Although a boon to veterans and workers, these programs also were an incentive to feign or exaggerate a problem to receive monetary benefits. Thus, several tests were developed or adapted to expose FEHL and to quantify hearing.

The special tests for FEHL were fairly reliable and valid but they became antiquated because of their inherent limitations and the rise of better audiometric procedures. EDA lost favor because some patients could not be conditioned, and there were ongoing ethical and legal concerns about shocking people. The D-S test was intricate and time consuming. The tone version of DAF was quite rapid and accurate, but some people could not consistently tap out the rhythm pattern even without delayed feedback. Békésy audiometry was helpful in detecting or confirming FEHL but not in indicating genuine hearing sensitivity. By the 1970s, electrophysiologic measures, mainly auditory brainstem response testing, supplanted all the previous procedures.

As part of the enormous interest in FEHL, there were attempts to discern characteristics of persons presenting unreliable and invalid results. Some of the tendencies reported were slightly lower intelligence, more psychiatric and psychosomatic complaints, less conformity to societal morality, less emotional stability, and lower income. Although those with FEHL generally had a less favorable profile, it is paramount to bear in mind that the differences in some dimensions were small and in other dimensions nonexistent.

The next chapter looks at the demographic elements of adults with FEHL, namely, prevalence, gender, age, and degree of supposed hearing loss. It also explores monetary and psychological phenomena that contribute to the genesis and maintenance of FEHL.

Chapter 3

ADULTS

Among the hundreds of patients with functional hearing loss whom I have seen, there were a number of instances in which there were demonstrable psychologic problems, as determined by psychologic or psychiatric evaluation, severe enough to account for all or part of the observed audiometric discrepancies.

—Ventry, 1968, p. 90

Introduction

It is appropriate to devote separate chapters to adults and children because in many ways their situations are not comparable. This chapter gives a synopsis of current knowledge about adults with FEHL and considers factors that contribute to the condition. The following chapter does much the same regarding children.

Characteristics of Adults with FEHL

The bulk of the literature on adults with FEHL in the past four decades has been on evaluation methods and on descriptions of group characteristics.

Prevalence-Incidence

As seen in Chapter 2, information on prevalence is clouded by several complicating factors, most notably an enormous ascertainment bias of the population reported on. Most reports in the postwar era had to do with military-industrial situations and potential compensation; although less so today, they still predominate. Although statistics are not kept on FEHL among military veterans, prevalence in veterans apparently decreased in the 1970s and 1980s (Rintelmann & Schwan, 1999). The military hearing conservation programs of the 1960s and 1970s were likely a main reason. In addition to greater attention to hearing protection, the programs had better instrumentation, tests, and testers, as well as longitudinal audiologic records. These may have militated against attempts to simulate a hearing loss (Rintelmann & Schwan, 1999). In the civilian arena, the Occupational and Safety Health Act (OSHA) of 1970 must have had similar effects for similar reasons. Such thorough programs probably would deter an individual from making a false claim and put the burden of proof on the employee that the employer was negligent.

In one review of 162 medicolegal cases, 116 were applying for workers' compensation (Barelli & Ruder, 1970). Of those, 24% had symptoms of FEHL. Gold, Hunsaker, and Haseman (1991) identified 18 military personnel as having FEHL out of more than 2100 audiologic evaluations (0.9%) in one year at a U.S. Naval hospital induction center. De Koker (2004) cited a 32% incidence rate of FEHL among 160 mine workers during a 3-month period in South Africa where there is potential compensation.

Nilo and Saunders (1976) found FEHL in 85 to 90% of 600 referrals from a military induction center but they found FEHL only "in more than 1 percent" in a general population. Without citing data, Jerger and Jerger (1981) believed the prevalence of FEHL was 10 to 50% among persons pursuing compensation but less than 2% in the general population. They felt that in an ordinary clinic one case a month of any age might appear. This agrees with the present author's review of 90 FEHL patients of all ages at a teaching medical center in 64 months (Peck, 2002). That corresponds to 1.4 cases per month or one case per 150 patients (0.9%). Rintelmann and Schwan (1999) also estimated a frequency of less than 2% among adults based on their experience in university, hospital, and private audiology centers. These agree with Qiu, Yin, Stucker, and Welsh's (1998) experience in an otolaryngology service at a teaching medical center. They identified 64 FEHL cases out of 4720 evaluations for a prevalence rate of 1.4%. Spraggs, Burton, and Graham (1994) reported that five patients being evaluated for a cochlear implant had better hearing than initially displayed as confirmed by electrophysiologic measurement of evoked responses; one had normal hearing. These five patients were less than 1% of their cases.

Gender and Age

Many reports since the end of the postwar era had to do with potential compensation. One may safely presume that most of those patients were male. In one series, all 18 military personnel were male (Gold, Hunsaker, & Haseman, 1991). At two general otolaryngology services, both genders were represented but there were contrasting findings. In one (Qiu et al., 1998), 45 of 64 patients were males (70%) and 19 were females (30%), yielding a ratio of 2.4:1 in favor of males. In the other, the ratio was nearly the reverse. Of 31 patients, 24 (77%) were female and 7 were male, a ratio 3.4:1 in favor of females (Hiraumi, Tsuji, Kanemaru, Fujino, & Ito, 2007). In the Peck (2002) series at a general teaching hospital, the sex makeup among the 29 adults was 19 female and 10 male or 2:1 female.

The average age of patients was 28 years in the Gold et al. (1991) report. Their patients ranged in age from 18 to 53 years. Peck's (2002) adult patients had an age span from 18 to 59 years. The overall average age was 34; females tended to be younger with an average age of 31 years versus the males' average age of 40 years. Holenweg and Kompis's (2010) 18 patients were similar with an age range of 19 to 57 years and an average of 40. Qiu et al.'s (1998) study did not separate children from adults for reporting purposes. The age range was 9 to 65 years with an average of 35 years.

Contrary to most literature of that era, the majority of Berk and Feldman's (1958) cases were not adults but children and adolescents. Moreover, the evidence showed that FEHL in children was underdiagnosed by otologists and audiologists because of lack of awareness. Reports that encompassed patients of all ages counted more children than adults. Peck's (2002) 90 cases consisted of only 29 adults as opposed to 61 children. Holenweg and Kompis (2010) found 18 adults versus 22 children.

Hearing Loss

Degree

Despite the many reports on adults with FEHL, statistics on the magnitude of false hearing losses are scarce. Peck (2002) could not calculate average hearing loss, because often thresholds were not obtained. To explain, as soon as results were suspect, intensity was kept low and not always increased to the point of an initial minimum response level. The only thing that could be said was that the range of initial hearing loss went from mild to no response. Holenweg and Kompis (2010) found that most of their FEHL patients portrayed hearing losses of 40 dB to 60 dB. Otherwise, magnitude of invalid hearing losses is hardly reported. Only rarely have there been reports of air-bone gaps or conductive losses, except as accompanied by an exaggeration.

One Versus Two Ears

There is no clear majority of FEHL presentations being for one ear or for two. Gold et al. (1991) came across 14 bilateral "losses" in 18 cases (78%). Hiraumi et al. (2007) reported finding 17 instances of bilateral and 14 of unilateral FEHL. Martin (2009), the audiologist who has, perhaps, devoted more attention to FEHL than any other in the past few decades, believes that bilateral cases are far and away in the majority. However, when Qiu et al. (1998) combined their entirely simulated cases and exaggerated cases, unilateral presentations outnumbered bilaterals 38 to 24. Their most common single class of FEHL was a simulated unilateral hearing loss (44% of all cases). Purely simulated losses, both uni- and bilateral, constituted 65% of the group, whereas 29% were exaggerated sensorineural hearing losses; only 6% had true conductive/mixed hearing losses. Peck's (2002) adult cases were evenly split at 14 bilateral and 15 unilateral instances.

Magnitude and Form of Overlay

Gelfand and Silman studied the size as well as the shape of false components. They assessed the difference between the false thresholds and the resolved thresholds. Their first study was of bilateral exaggerations (63 patients) (Gelfand & Silman, 1985), and their next experiment was of unilateral exaggerations in bilateral organic hearing losses (25 patients) (Gelfand & Silman, 1993). The configuration of the false component was related to the configuration of the true hearing levels. For normal hearing or mild impairments, the size of the overlay was consistent across frequencies. In cases with normal hearing followed by a true precipitous high-frequency drop, the overlay was dramatically smaller at the impaired frequencies. Cases with moderate or severe sloping losses were in between, that is, the false portion became gradually smaller with increasing frequency. However, there was wide intersubject variability in both the false and the true hearing losses. Keeping that in mind, the average size of the false component was 25 to 40 dB for low- and mid-frequencies and was 20 dB or less for severe high-frequency losses.

Gelfand (1993) analyzed overlays in a novel way by having subjects with sensorineural losses exaggerate their hearing losses. Again, configurations of the false components varied with frequency. The differences in size and shape of the overlays were associated with: (a) normal hearing, (b) abrupt losses at 4000 Hz, and (c) sloping losses, respectively. The data from the experimental subjects substantiated the findings obtained from clinical patients, whose false components had resolved. Gelfand and Silman considered the results of all three studies to be consistent with a patient strategy of using an internal loudness target, or "anchor," on a within-ear basis. The anchor concept also fitted with the effect of loudness recruitment in that the false components were smaller where the impairments were sizable.

Several generalizations can be made about adult FEHL, but given the limited information, they should be viewed with caution. There is a wide range of reported prevalence/incidence. The prevalence reported in compensation situations is uneven at 10 to 45%, but there is fairly good agreement on a prevalence of 1% in noncompensation situations. The great preponderance of patients in compensation cases are males. In contrast, in general settings females may be more prevalent by 2:1. The proportion of bilateral versus unilateral presentation is unclear but there are probably more bilateral cases. The range of alleged hearing losses is wide. The hearing losses appear overwhelmingly as sensorineural. The age span is from young adulthood to about 60 years, and most of the adults are in their 20s to 40s.

Causal, Contributing, and Maintaining Factors

Monetary Incentives

A major cause of FEHL in adults is the opportunity for financial gain from feigning a hearing loss. Indeed, the greater the disability, the greater is the benefit. Given human nature, when there is the chance to acquire money by making hearing appear worse than it is, some people will do so, especially if money cannot be easily obtained otherwise (Noble, 1978).

An interesting speculation is whether economic conditions influence the rate of false health complaints or hearing test behaviors, as Nilo and Saunders (1976) supposed. This author sought information by writing several university economists. Eight professors from five institutions replied that it was an interesting question; although they thought that such a link was possible, even likely, none knew of any literature on the question. However, one economist cited a study showing, counterintuitively, that claims of back pain increased during prosperous periods and decreased during recessionary periods (Brooker, Frank, & Tarasuk, 1997). In any event, attempts to find information specific to the relationship between false claims and economic conditions have not been fruitful, so it remains an open question.

Psychological Influences

This section looks at psychological influences in FEHL. The falsification categories, themselves, of malingering, factitious disorder, and conversion disorder are covered in Chapter 10 on psychosocial considerations. Individuals might falsely present a hearing loss for subtler reasons than monetary gain or frank conversion disorder. They may, with varying degrees of intent, seek other benefits (e.g., an explanation for lack of career advancement or for poor personal adjustment). Moreover, if and how they present a hearing loss is influenced by numerous factors.

> There is a subtle interplay between organic factors causing physical injury and functional factors such as personality type, pre-existing psychiatric disease or vulnerability, substance misuse, gender, employment status, legal framework, unrelated but coincidental life events and related life events such as ill health retirement, conscious and unconscious exaggeration and the effects of litigation. (Thomas, 2002, p. 392)

A persistent issue in psychophysiological conditions is: Why does a particular symptom appear instead of another? In the context of this book, the question is, "Why hearing loss?" Presumably, some incident directed attention, consciously or otherwise, to the ears, such as infection, injury, exposure to very loud sound, hearing loss in a relative, or even hearing terribly painful words (Monsell & Herzon, 1984).

Compensation Neurosis

Sometimes mentioned in discussions of deception is "compensation neurosis," the exaggerated symptoms presented after an accident or injury when there is the prospect of financial compensation (Colman, 2001). For the most part, the term has fallen out of use. Using standard criteria of diagnostic validity, "compensation neurosis," does not measure up to a distinct disorder (Mendelson, 1985), and it is not listed as a disorder in the DSM-IV-TR. For that matter, "neurosis" is no longer a mainstream term in psychiatry. In spite of this, Hutchinson (2001) avers that compensation neurosis is a legitimate and complex syndrome, like the other disorders of simulation, malingering and factitious disorder. In other words, the deception is not motivated simply by monetary compensation.

Comorbidity

Comorbidity is the coexistence of two or more disorders that may or may not influence each other, usually one of them being considered the primary disorder. Coexisting disorders could be of any sort—mental, perceptual, neurological, and so on—and they do not have to be organic. The significance is that one disorder could facilitate the adopting of another. Based on the above literature, this author's experience, and information about children in the next chapter, it seems likely that many persons with FEHL have comorbid conditions. Some case reports later in the chapter are illustrative.

Symptom Perception and Psychological State

Beliefs and feelings about a symptom influence how it is experienced. Thus, how bad the symptom seems is not in a direct one-to-one relationship with the degree of actual injury. By being overly preoccupied about a particular symptom, the sufferer may feel it disproportionately. A person who is fixated on the hearing loss may present, unintentionally, greater loss than actually exists or may complain excessively about the severity (Main, 2003).

A false overlay could stem from worry that a genuine hearing loss would jeopardize job security, or that hearing could worsen or already was getting worse. A person could then behave in everyday life as if he or she actually had that degree of hearing impairment. Furthermore, that person might subconsciously take a hearing test in a way that is compatible with their believed hearing loss (Beagley & Knight, 1968; Coles, 1993).

If an individual is so troubled by the circumstances surrounding the onset of the symptom, the symptom can be magnified or perpetuated. This might happen following a physical trauma incurred during a highly upsetting event, such as a serious work injury or an assault. Such a physical trauma often is also an emotional or psychological trauma. A relevant example is a female struck on the ear by a male during an altercation. The blow may or may not have caused bleeding or pain, and so on, but the frightening circumstances, themselves, help create the sense of hearing loss or cause its perpetuation or magnification (see Bagby, Wild, & Turner, 2003). As a clinical note, a female with a perforation of the left tympanic membrane is a red flag of having been assaulted, because most people are right handed.

Another dynamic is exaggerating when patients are concerned about not being believed (Main, 2003). They may have been told that their problem was imaginary or "all in your head." They may feel it is necessary to exaggerate to make sure that the problem is unmistakable to convince evaluators, family, co-workers, and so on that the situation is real. They may not even be aware of exaggerating.

All of these influences may move some people unintentionally to overreport their symptoms or exaggerate their degree of dysfunction. Such exaggeration is more likely in persons who are seriously depressed, or who have a personality or somatoform disorder (see Bagby, Wild, & Turner, 2003). An audiologist probably would not know if a particular patient had such a disorder, which should make clinicians more sensitive to patients with exaggerated results. In summary, a person's anxiety about their hearing—impaired nor not—can trigger, help maintain, or magnify a FEHL.

Formal studies of psychosocial adjustment have been lacking over the decades. One clinical report (Peck, 2002) described findings on 90 patients of all ages with FEHL. Peck interviewed the patients about factors that could have contributed to obtaining uncertain results. (Approaches to interviewing about sensitive issues are discussed in Chapter 11, Management.) Many patients did express substantial apprehension about some aspect of their lives. In a number of cases, a highly disturbing event had occurred around the time of the onset of the "hearing loss." Based on their reports, Peck considered 14 of 29 (48%) adult patients at risk of having a psychosocial disorder.

Context: Test Versus Nontest Situation

Noble (1978, 1987) considers the context of the evaluation itself a main cause of false test results. Malingerers feign a hearing loss only in the clinical setting, but persons with a conversion disorder behave as though hearing impaired in and out of the test setting. One may wonder if the division is always so complete.

As Noble sees it, a person with little income who wants to increase it can fake a hearing loss on a test and acquire money. The person does not have a psychiatric disorder, just not much money, and faking is simply a shrewd way to get more income, maybe the only way the person has. The faker is engaging in a dishonest act but of a rather minor degree, in Noble's view. Cheaters are "*doing* something wrong, but *have* nothing wrong with them" (Noble, 1987, p. 2).

Noble calls this element of hearing testing "*fakability*," that is, how easy and inviting it is to fake test results. He deems the problem not as much with the person as with the process, which involves the use of "inadequate tests" that are so fakable.

Noble's 1978 book is a refreshing, unconventional, and thought-provoking look at the entire field of hearing assessment, and is well-reasoned with much support from an extensive literature. This author sees merit in Noble's "fakability" construct. However, this author's view is that faking often goes beyond not having much money to include an element of greed, that is, some fakers are not so economically disadvantaged but see a chance at easy money. Also, Noble's view seems to put the burden of wrongdoing on the system rather on the person who is acting dishonestly.

Deaf Wannabee

There is a group of people, who not only want to appear deaf, but who truly want to be deaf or take on the lifestyle of a deaf person. This is not in the sense of malingering or of a conversion or classic factitious disorder. According to the Deaf Wannabee (2008) Web site, the underlying reason is a sexual fetish about hearing aids or deafness. People might want to be deaf for a variety of reasons, such as feeling that they are deaf people stuck in a hearing body (perhaps somewhat like persons who are transsexual feeling they are in the wrong sex body). Their Web site offers advice on how to deafen oneself either temporarily or permanently. They are fiercely protective of their right to want to be deaf. This segment of society must be exceedingly small and, indeed, be a very small proportion of persons who falsely claim hearing impairment or take on the life of a severely hearing-impaired person. As such, they constitute a variant of the usual idea of FEHL.

Sample Cases of FEHL

Case 1

PM, a 34-year-old female, came to the ENT clinic complaining of hearing loss in her right ear since sinus surgery a week ago. She also complained of headaches and blurry vision. She did not respond to pure tones in her right ear up to 40 dB and gave scattered responses to left-ear signals at 40 dB. However, she followed conversation at 30 dB, and SRT words were familiarized at 30 dB. Initial SRTs were 20 dB. PM leaned forward and strained to hear much of the time. She often said "a little bit" in time with a tone stimulus. Finally, after reinstructing a few times and coaxing, she passed a screening in each at 15 dB HL for 250 to 4000 Hz, and final SRTs were 15 dB. Afterward, she was told that her hearing was normal. In discussion with her, she denied stress but then described herself as very nervous. She had had stomach discomforts daily for years and pain in her side, each without explanation. She graduated from high school with low grades and was unemployed. She divulged that she had reduced libido for many years. She was agreeable to seeking mental health evaluation. It would seem safe to say that even a person without psychological training would deduce that PM was quite anxious, likely had low mood, was economically precarious, and that her false hearing loss and other symptoms were interconnected (comorbidity).

Case 2

LH, a 54-year-old female, was referred from the ENT clinic because a Weber tuning fork test was referred to the left ear and she had had surgery for neck cancer a year ago. Initial results suggested a 70-dB hearing loss in the right ear with little air-bone gap, unmasked. SRTs were 20 dB in each ear. Her word recognition scores at 10 dB SL (30 dB HL) were 94%. Final pure-tone "thresholds" suggested a flat

25 dB hearing loss, which probably was poorer than her true hearing. She was reassured that her hearing turned out to be fine. LH acknowledged difficulty concentrating since cancer surgery the year before, a difficulty which her relatives had also noticed. Her father died about a year ago, and she was not getting over it as one should, in her opinion, or as she did when her mother died. She did not enjoy her grandchildren as she used to. For the past year, she lost her voice completely by the end of each work day, even though her job did not require talking. She disclosed that she was depressed. It seems obvious that this woman was very troubled. Within the past year, she experienced the devastating loss of her father, had a life-threatening illness of her own requiring major surgery, was unhappy, and inexplicably lost her voice daily (likely a comorbid symptom with her emotional burdens). There seemed to be more than sufficient basis for referral to a mental health care provider. Indeed, not suggesting referral could have been considered a disservice. These findings were discussed with the otolaryngologist, who concurred with the referral. LH agreed that counseling was in order.

Case 3

BP, a 23-year-old male, had been in a motor vehicle crash. His right ear had been lacerated and sutured and he had bled from the ear canal. He also had injuries to the left shoulder, ribs, and hip, and there was a presumed basilar skull fracture. An audiologic evaluation at 9 days suggested a 70-dB pure-tone hearing loss in the right ear but better hearing for speech. Hearing was re-evaluated 9 days later. Results reliably showed a 60-dB loss in the right ear and a mild loss in rising configuration in the left ear. However, the pure tone Stenger test was positive, suggesting a 23-dB exaggeration on the right side, and he responded to speech in the right ear well below the pure-tone results. After urging and discussing, his responses to right-ear signals improved to the point of passing a 20-dB screening, except for a 40-dB 4000-Hz notch loss. SRTs were at least as low as 15 dB. Word recognition scores at 10-dB SL were 92% in the right ear and 100% in the left ear. The impression was normal hearing in both ears with the exception of the right-ear, high-frequency notch. The mother was with the audiologist in the control booth observing. She thought that there was a "psychological component" to his recovery from the frightening event. BP said that his left leg and ribs still hurt, which limited his activity, and he felt he had a hearing loss in his right ear, even though he and his mother agreed that it did not cause a communication problem. It appears highly unlikely that this is a case of malingering. Rather, it seems to represent comorbid physical injuries and symptom over-reaction related to ear bleeding and suturing and the overall physical and psychological trauma of the incident.

Case 4

DA, a 25-year-old male, was referred for thorough evaluation because of inconsistent test results elsewhere. He reported that he sustained a hearing loss in his right ear because of a work-related blow to that ear. The test a week earlier had suggested a severe hearing loss in the right ear, but responses were inconsistent. DA wanted a hearing test for his attorney for possible litigation. The patient responded consistently during testing of the left ear and showed normal hearing for pure tones and speech. When testing the right ear, there was no response at equipment maximum. The absence of a crossover response showed invalid performance. Despite reinstructing, responses did not improve; however, he answered an offhand question to the right ear at 50 dB HL. The pure-tone and speech Stenger tests were positive. Minimum contralateral interference levels for tones came at 15 to 30 dB HL and for spondees at 22 dB HL. Because the level to the left ear was 10 dB SL, it was reasoned that genuine thresholds in the right ear were about 10 dB better than the Stenger interference levels, which would mean normal sensitivity at 20 dB or better. Repeat evaluation was recommended. Nowhere during the discussion or in the report was the word or notion of "malingering" brought up, even though this appears to be a case of knowingly fabricating a hearing loss for compensation. DA undoubtedly had a job injury, which could have impaired hearing temporarily. Nevertheless, there is little point in an audiologist speculating on the degree of intentionality, and it is possible that there could be some symptom perpetuation.

Pseudo-pseudohypacusis, Obscure Auditory Dysfunction

On rare occasion audiologists see patients who credibly complain of hearing difficulty yet are easily tested by conventional audiometry, display normal hearing, and have no signs or risk factors for FEHL. Because these patients have no explanatory history and understand speech quite well in the interview, a clinician might be suspicious that the claim of hearing trouble was false. However, finding normal hearing so easily is not at all the typical way people present a false hearing impairment. In other words, they might give the false impression of false hearing loss, a situation this author has only somewhat facetiously dubbed pseudo-pseudohypacusis.

In this writer's experience, these individuals are unquestionably having difficulty understanding speech. They tend to be young adults, female, and achievement-oriented with high self-expectations. Their complaint extends back a few months or years, and, upon closer interview, arose during a difficult time in their lives. A pattern typically emerges of a person who feels considerable stress, expects much of him- or herself and of others, and knows or supposes that others have high expectations of them, too. Some of these patients also are dealing with considerable sadness. When told that their hearing sensitivity is normal, they tend to be relieved but confused, because they are most definitely encountering difficulties. Pains are taken to assure the patient that the clinician does not disbelieve the complaints and that finding normal hearing (pure-tone sensitivity) does not mean that there is no problem. When this audiologist reflects to patients that some such individuals often have a "preoccupation" that is interfering with efficient listening, they are surprised yet express an awakening realization or outright admission of some deep concern. When the idea is raised of conferring with a person in the field of mental health, there is acceptance and even gratitude and relief.

Saunders and Haggard (1989) noticed a puzzling triad of difficulty understanding speech in noise, normal pure-tone thresholds, and lack of a cause of the difficulty, which they named "obscure auditory dysfunction" (OAD). OAD is a multifactorial syndrome with auditory, psychological, and linguistic components. Cause and prevalence are uncertain, although Stephens, Zhao, and Kennedy (2003) claimed that this condition occurs in 5 to 10% of those going to clinics complaining of hearing problems. The age range is 15 to 55 years with an average of 31 years. The female-male ratio is 2:1, and educational level is above average (Saunders, Field, & Haggard, 1992). Most first notice their problem in the preceding 3 years. Saunders and colleagues found that patients with OAD had more than average difficulty on tests of understanding speech in noise as well as a raised degree of anxiety, but that OAD does not comprise a homogeneous group (Saunders & Haggard, 1992, 1993). The condition may be linked to minor peripheral or central auditory dysfunction, and often those affected show evidence of anxious or depressive personalities (Stephens, Zhao, & Kennedy, 2003). They believe they cannot hear as well as others when, in fact, they can (Saunders & Forsline, 2006; Saunders, Forsline, & Fausti, 2004). Saunders agrees that the patients' belief that their hearing ought to be better fits with the present writer's observation that some patients are self-demanding, high achievers (G. Saunders, personal communication, December 12, 2007).

This author is unsure whether the approximately 10 patients in his experience had OAD, although they certainly seem to have many of the characteristics. Two features stand out to this audiologist. First is the significance of life circumstances found in most of those patients. The second feature is the absence of symptoms or signs of auditory difficulty in the first two decades of life, specifically, academic difficulty or unusual trouble understanding in noise. Regardless of the diagnostic category, these people definitely need proper management.

Sample Cases of Pseudo-pseudohypacusis

Case 1

A man in his 40s was experiencing difficulty understanding speech in the past year. He had a somewhat flat affect. Pure-tone audiometry promptly showed normal sensitivity. The audiologist used the ploy of suggesting that, when we are preoccupied with what is going on inside, we are less available for what's coming in from outside. The audiologist gently inquired as to other aspects of his life, and out came his unhappy situation. His son had died many years previous. As he put it, he could not move past it. He had valiantly suppressed thoughts of sadness, not wanting to succumb to grief and feel the terrible pain and loss and thereby be impaired in his usual life affairs. His depressed mood was getting worse. He had no fun. He and wife used to enjoy outings and company, but no longer do so. When it was suggested that his notable attempts to keep from being overwhelmed might be preventing him from going through a grief process, he sullenly agreed. He was teary and acknowledged that he had not moved on. He readily accepted the thought that counseling was advisable. He was relieved that his situation made sense and felt good about leaving with the hope that he will not always have to feel so bad. As he was departing, he expressed much gratitude and looked and sounded better.

Case 2

JL, a third-year medical student, was having trouble understanding speech for a couple of years. She could not understand in surgery with everyone wearing masks, and she missed conversation while walking with friends, when no one else did. The previous year had been "horrible." Some friends had attempted suicide. Her father was gravely ill. She vomited every morning, but a gastrointestinal consult was negative. Pure-tone audiometry easily showed normal sensitivity. It was pointed out that hearing difficulty despite normal hearing is most often seen in young females who are high achievers. "That is certainly me!" she said. As with the above patient, the audiologist used phraseology about being preoccupied with things inside. She asked, "Could stress affect your hearing?" She was told that it could affect performance. She launched into organic and medical thinking. "I had psychiatry. I don't think I have a personality disorder. I know about somatoform disorders." As the examiner said that people respond differently to stress, tears welled up. Then, her first insight: "I'm starting to see this pattern of stresses and all." At times, JL dissolved into painful tears. When the idea was suggested of discussing these things with a specialist, she said, "You mean like counseling?" More tears. Eventually, she indicated that she would talk to an admired physician in student health.

Case 3

AH was a prospective medical student. For a few years, he needed people to repeat to him more often than is usual. In earning his college degree and his master's in engineering, hearing had not been an impediment. During pure-tone audiometry, he promptly responded to all tones at 0 to 5 dB HL. Afterward, the clinician mentioned the notion that being preoccupied with something can make it harder to listen effectively. He was asked if that might apply. Life had been smooth until a year ago, when his fiancée broke their engagement. He had planned to enter the military but could not, which was a big disappointment. He felt highly stressed working as a lab assistant while hoping to be accepted into medical school. He had frequent, unexplained bowel symptoms. The audiologist used the tactic of describing some symptoms found in persons who question their hearing but have normal sensitivity. Suddenly, he exclaimed in distress, "You gotta stop. You're describing me!" He was accepting and comfortable with the suggestion to see someone in mental health.

Summary

As best can be surmised, the prevalence of adult FEHL is one percent in a general population seeking hearing assessment and 10 to 45% in compensation cases. Most of those displaying FEHL are males, at least in situations involving remuneration, but, conversely, most persons in such remunerative situations are male. Whether bilateral presentations are more common than unilateral presentations is likely but not firmly established. There is no typical age, but the majority of patients are between 20 and 40 years old.

In addition to the opportunity to obtain money, psychological matters help initiate, maintain, or magnify FEHL. Psychological factors include a coexisting mental or physical disorder (comorbidity); excessive preoccupation about impact on life and livelihood; fear of disbelief by others; and distressing circumstances surrounding the onset of the supposed hearing loss. Perhaps, our evaluation procedures are too "fakable," too easily falsified and thereby contribute to FEHL. A very small segment of society (Deaf Wannabees) takes on the life of a hearing impaired person for psychosexual reasons and constitutes a rare variant of FEHL.

Finally, there is a subset of patients who have genuine difficulty understanding speech in noise but also have normal findings on standard auditory tests, and do not have any form of FEHL ("pseudo-pseudohypacusis"). Some may have an obscure auditory dysfunction. Several factors might be in play: a challenging time in their life, high expectations, feelings of stress or sadness, minor peripheral or central auditory dysfunction, and underestimation of their hearing ability.

Now that we have considered the area of adults with FEHL, the next chapter addresses children. A number of differences between the two age groups are evident, and audiologists need to be aware of them.

Chapter 4

CHILDREN

Psychological problems can be detected through hearing screening tests, which, in many cases, have been the only method by which a psychological problem has been discovered.

—Berk and Feldman, 1958, p. 216

Introduction

There are similarities between adults and children with FEHL but also significant differences. Some of the differences involve history, causes, motives, and life issues, not to mention evaluation techniques and management, which are discussed in later chapters. This chapter covers information about children with FEHL.

Characteristics of Children with FEHL

Prevalence

If reports of prevalence-incidence among adults were tenuous, the matter is worse with children. Opinions that false hearing loss among children "is not rare" go back 50 years (Barr, 1960; Dixon & Newby, 1959). Since then, several authors have asserted that childhood FEHL is "not uncommon" or is "more common than supposed," whatever that may be (Pracy, Walsh, Mepham, & Bowdler, 1996). Despite the lack of empirical data, this author agrees with these assertions. On the other hand, reports that do mention incidence are fairly compatible. Out of 1900 children in a school hearing screening program, Leshin (1960) found 2.5% showing signs of FEHL. Pracy et al. (1996) put their incidence at about a 1% in a year. Peck (2002) and Saravanappa, Mepham, and Bowdler (2005) encountered about 1 case per 150 patients of all ages (0.9% incidence), or nearly one a month. Campanelli (1963) found 41 children in a total caseload at an audiology clinic of 2300 or 1.7% of a group seen in 1 year. Barr's (1963) incidence rate was three or four cases per year.

Childhood FEHL often has a rapid beginning but is not obvious to others. The onset is not marked by alarm on the part of the patient, as it is in genuine hearing loss. Sudden true hearing loss is a rare pathology in children. Hence, Psarommatis, Kontorinis, Kontrogiannis, Douniadakis, and Tsakanikos (2009) evaluated the incidence of false hearing loss in children who presented with sudden hearing loss. They reviewed the medical records of 48 children seen in a 5-year period, who underwent comprehensive medical and audiologic evaluation, including testing for otoacoustic emissions. In 26 patients, or 54%, the hearing losses were false. The authors asserted that "pseudohypacusis" represents the most frequent explanation for sudden hearing loss in children. Incidentally, the total of 22 patients who had genuine organic hearing loss corresponds to about 4 cases per year, which attests to the relative rarity of sudden hearing loss in children.

Gender and Age

There is a consistent, substantial predominance of girls by about two to one (Table 4–1). Based on the number of boys and girls in the various reports, this author calculated the gender ratios to range from 1.5:1 to 3.5:1 in favor of girls. The average age is 11 years, and the age span is from 6 to 18 years.

Hearing Loss

Children present a large variation in degree of false hearing loss from mild to severe. The supposed hearing loss involves both ears far more often than one ear. The audiometric configurations vary but most are flat or resemble a curve of most comfortable listening level for normal hearers (Lehrer et al., 1964; Yoshida, Noguchi, & Uemura, 1989). Another area of great unanimity is that there rarely is an air-bone gap. Not surprisingly, it was frequently reported that thresholds for speech were better than for pure tones (Barr, 1960; Pracy et al., 1996).

Clinicians have been impressed by how well children follow conversation when they do not feel they are being tested, which is a very typical clue to FEHL (Lehrer et al., 1964; Pracy et al., 1996). Resolving false results is easier with children than with adults. Many hearing "losses" improve to normal hearing levels with no difficulty or with mild encouragement or reinstruction (Klotz, Koch, & Hackett,

Table 4–1. Summary of Childhood FEHL as to Gender, Age, Uni– or Bilateral, and Degree of Professed Loss

Study	*N*	*Female/ Male*		*Avg. Age*	*Age Range*	*No. Bilat. (%)*	*Avg. Loss*	*Loss Range*
Aplin and Rowson (1986, 1990)	30	20	10	12	7–16	30 (100%)	40	40–70 great majority
Barr (1963)	32	—	—	—	—	32 (100%)	—	60–80
Bowdler and Rogers (1989)	15	10	5	11	7–16	15 (100%)	58	—
Campanelli (1963)	41	27	14	11	6–17	35 (85%)	55	35–75 majority
Dixon and Newby (1959)	40	31	9	11	6–18	—	—	50–70 dB
Holenweg and Kompis (2010)	22	14	8	11	7–16	20 (90%)	50	30–80 most
Lehrer et al. (1964)	10	—	—	—	11–16	9 (90%)	—	35–85
McCanna and DeLapa (1981)	27	16	11	—	6–15	27 (100%)	—	—
Morita et al. (2010)	47	33	14	9	6–18	29 (62%)	—	65
Peck (2002)	61	42	19	11	7–17	44 (73%)	—	mild to NR
Pracy et al. (1996)	10	6	4	12	—	10 (100%)	51	—
Radkowski et al. (1998)	18	14	4	—	5–21	12 (67%)	—	—
Yoshida et al. (1989)	39	27	12	—	—	32 (82%)	—	mild–moderate

1960). By and large, parents have not noticed that their children acted hearing impaired, perhaps until learning the results of a school hearing screening. Table 4–1 summarizes the literature on childhood FEHL as to demographics and to alleged hearing loss.

Psychosocial Background

In contrast to the situation with adults, numerous reports regarding children deal with psychosocial conditions. Several terms overlap with psychosocial, especially as they apply to a disorder: emotional, mental, psychological, and psychiatric. (Indeed, some definitions include the name of one of the other disorders.) These terms may not be synonymous but they have common elements: (a) distressing thoughts or feelings, and (b) behaviors or symptoms that impair functioning in usual activities or that hinder maintaining relationships. Different sources use different terms, but they seem to be used interchangeably.

Writing as a psychologist in a child psychiatry journal, Broad (1980) reviewed papers from the late 1940s that dealt with the supposed symbolic significance of the ear and hearing. Although outdated, the thinking of the time gives a remarkably different, yet valuable, look at hearing as a defense against hurting or unacceptable words and sounds. Children with FEHL present "the picture of a painful early childhood which is dealt with through the massive use of denial and repression" (Broad, 1980, p. 52). They show poor self-concept, low self-esteem, great sensitivity to criticism, and poor ability to deal with peers; in essence, they see the world as a dangerous and potentially annihilating place. False hearing loss acts as a sort of gatekeeper that protects a fragile sense of self.

Some chilling reports show the protective function of "hearing loss." An 11-year-old girl who developed FEHL had a mentally ill father (Berk & Feldman, 1958). She tried to hide under a pillow and block her ears so she would not have to hear his screaming and other "emotionally loaded situations in her hearing environment that were threatening to her psychological balance and eventually caused her to block them out auditorily" (Berk & Feldman, 1958, p. 216).

Lumio, Jauhiainen, and Gelhar (1969) described a horrible family situation in which the father was violent toward the mother and the children. The youngest daughter, age 9 years, began to lose hearing; a few months later, her sisters complained of hearing and vision difficulty. After another several months, while away from home, the girls' hearing and vision returned to normal in one day. The authors ascribed the hearing loss (and low vision) to family turmoil.

Yet another disturbing example of "psychogenic deafness" was an 8-year-old boy in a terrible family situation, who suddenly developed hearing loss in his left ear (Chawla, Handa, & Tripathi, 2007). His mother had committed suicide, and his sister had been sent to boarding school. The father remarried, and the boy felt that the stepmother was more caring and loving toward his half brothers. Four days after being threatened with being sent away to school if he did not do well on an examination, the patient complained of hearing loss and could not take the exam. Pure-tone audiometry showed profound left-sided hearing loss, yet his auditory brainstem response was normal. Psychological tests showed emotional and interpersonal difficulties and fear of abandonment. The patient was treated alone with supportive therapy, and the parents were helped to understand the child's psychological situation and the need for a warm and loving environment. After 2 months of regular follow-ups, hearing returned completely.

Ahead of their time, Berk and Feldman (1958) opined that childhood FEHL, even if malingered, was based on underlying psychological needs. Because hearing screenings are a main source of referral for audiologic evaluation, they can be the first step in uncovering a psychological problem. They put forth the striking idea that hearing testing might be the only method by which a child's psychological problem comes to light.

Symptoms

The list of symptoms among children with FEHL is wide-ranging. One study found feelings of insecurity, inadequacy, hostility, tension, anxiety, and aggression (Lehrer et al., 1964). On a personality inventory of children having FEHL, the most salient personality characteristics were introversion or a combination of introversion and neuroticism, especially in girls (Aplin & Rowson, 1986). Only 20% were within normal limits on all dimensions of the inventory. Cases with deeper psychological problems tended to present greater hearing loss. Most of Dixon and Newby's (1959) 40 patients did not have noticeable emotional problems. However, in several instances, parents reported that their child had strong sibling rivalry, persistent enuresis, anxiety reactions, and a lack of satisfactory academic progress. McCanna and DeLapa (1981) stated that two thirds of their cases were either being followed by a psychologist or were described by their parents as being "nervous, easily upset, having peer-problems, experiencing sibling rivalry, being withdrawn, or having a disorganized personality" (McCanna & DeLapa, 1981, p. 27). With the help of the school psychologist and cooperation of the parents, follow-up a year later of 17 of the children found that they had passed their school hearing screening.

False visual symptoms were mentioned by Dixon and Newby (1959) and Lumio, Jauhiainen, and Gelhar (1969). Six of 18 of Radkowski, Cleveland, and Friedman's (1998) patients had failed school vision screenings and were found to have normal ophthalmologic examinations and vision.

Brooks and Geohegan (1993) looked at long-term outcome of 29 subjects who had displayed FEHL 6 to 27 years earlier. Five were or had been under psychiatric care. They concluded that FEHL may "indicate underlying problems" that call for further evaluation and therapy

Peck (2002) reported on his experience with 90 unselected patients, who displayed FEHL at a general teaching hospital. Sixty-one of the patients were children. The audiologist spoke separately with the child and with the accompanying adult, and then the two together. They were told that obtaining the test results had been more difficult than usual, and that sometimes that happened when a person was bothered by something in their lives. They were asked if that could apply in their case or if they if they had an idea as to possible causes. In addition, general questions were asked regarding how things were going with school, friends, and family or if anything was causing excessive "preoccupation." For some of the children aged 6 to 12 years, parents completed the Pediatric Symptom Checklist (PSC) (Jellinek et al., 1988). The PSC is a standardized, simple, pass-fail checklist to screen for psychosocial dysfunction (sensitivity, 0.95; specificity, 0.68).

Many times, care providers acknowledged that their child began to exhibit some negative behaviors in the previous year or so. In several instances, a traumatic event had occurred during that year, such as a family move, divorce, or death. A number of parents reported that their child had been sexually abused or substantial suspicion that such abuse had occurred. Based on the interviews, 40 of the 61 children were deemed at risk of having a psychosocial disorder. For 31 children within the age range of the PSC, 23 (74%) were at risk for such disorder. The clinical impression was that 20 of those 23 children were at risk. Conversely, the PSC suggested that 8 children (26%) were not at risk, and the clinical opinion agreed in 7 instances. Altogether, the clinical impressions and the PSC results coincided in 27 of 31 cases or 87% of the time.

Circumstantial Factors

Fifteen of 24 children (62%) in the McCanna and DeLapa (1981) series came from broken homes; many were living with persons who were not their parents. In several instances, parental divorce and remarriage and resultant change in home or school occurred just prior to the appearance of the false hearing loss.

Two other diagnostic cues need mentioning. Abuse has been found among children who display false hearing loss (Drake, Makielski, McDonald-Bell, & Atcheson, 1995; Riedner & Efros, 1995). When a child is found presenting an invalid hearing loss, abuse must be considered. Trauma is the other cue. Radkowski, Cleveland, and Friedman (1998) identified some preceding physical traumatic incident in 10 of their 18 young patients. The trauma took various forms: a teacher tugging on an ear, a football tackle, ototoxic chemotherapy, and, in seven cases, a history of acute otitis media including some having had ear surgery. In any event, a new hearing loss should prompt asking about recent ailment or injury.

Children with FEHL often are in situations of turmoil. In addition to difficult relations with peers and family discord, they are more likely to have had a sudden change in family dynamics, such as a new baby, a serious illness, or separation from an important figure through divorce, parental parting, or death (Mehta & Martindale, 2005). Based on experience, this writer would add to the list of sources of separation the death of a beloved person or pet, the move of a cherished friend to another locale, and the absence of one parent when the parents never married. Children often were wounded and bitter about the unmarried father not appearing for major holidays or events.

Intelligence and School Performance

Seventy-percent of Aplin and Rowson's (1986) patients either had school or home problems or both, as did seven of Bowdler and Rogers' (1989) 15 cases. By and large, children with FEHL have shown normal or only slightly low intelligence, yet they do not perform well in school. Four of Barr's (1960) 32 patients were designated as slightly mentally deficient. The mean verbal and performance IQs in Aplin and Rowson's (1990) sample were nearly identical and slightly below average at about 95, although there was a broad range of intellectual ability. Lehrer et al.'s (1964) 10 cases had a mean IQ of 89.

Supposed Causes of Childhood FEHL

Throughout decades of literature, a few factors are invariably repeated as being causes of childhood FEHL, namely, a drop in school performance, a history of middle ear disease, seeking attention, and psychological distress. They are accepted because they seem obvious and logical. Yet, with the exception of psychological distress, there is no evidence to support the relationships. This does not mean these conditions are extraneous. Following are several commonly believed causes of childhood FEHL for which there is no empirical corroboration.

Drop in School Performance

A drop in school performance is time and again cited as the basis of false hearing loss because it is often found in FEHL children and because it is a handy excuse readily accepted by parents (Aplin & Rowson, 1990; McCanna & DeLapa, 1981). Indeed, when one encounters a child with FEHL, school work usually is not going well, which fits the assumption that poor grades can lead to FEHL. However, inferring a causal relationship seems based on supposition and not on data. Correlation does not imply causation. In most patients, there is a rather definite time period when grades declined, which coincided with both a disturbing life event and the onset of the supposed hearing loss. If a child were experiencing some disturbing situation in life, it is quite reasonable to expect school performance to suffer. Given that children with FEHL are at risk for substantial emotional problems, it seems equally, if not more, likely, that both the lowered school achievement and the FEHL are co-symptoms of some other root factor.

Ear Disease

The idea that ear disease has a predisposing influence in FEHL sounds reasonable. A history of middle ear disorder affords first-hand experience with an ear problem (Aplin & Rowson, 1986, 1990; Lehrer et al., 1964). A child might perpetuate or adopt a hearing loss because of supposed benefits experienced at the time of having an ear problem, such as sympathy or being excused from chores (Pracy et al., 1996). Indeed, many children who display FEHL have had some ear problem. Again, however, correlation does not imply causation. Even though the incidence of otitis media drops off sharply in the first 4 years of life, it is not a rarity up to age 12. (Statistics on incidence by year after age 4 years are surprisingly lacking.) It is not unusual to find an 11-year-old child who had had otitis media at some point since starting school. Conversely, the great preponderance of children with a background of otitis media do not exhibit FEHL. There is little or no evidence that children who have had genuine hearing loss or ear disorder are more likely than other children to feign a hearing loss. Although having experienced an ear disorder may play a part in symptom selection, if clinicians focus on past ear problems, they may be misled and their attention diverted from considering a deeper hidden cause of a false hearing loss.

Mimicking

Supposedly, some children see the "benefit" that others derive from failing a hearing screening or from developing a hearing loss, so they mimic the condition to get the same benefits. However, most children do not want to be different. They do not like being singled out, or to go to the school nurse or other authority figure. They might not mind missing school, but they typically do not want to miss after-school activities or go to a physician, where there is the prospect of getting a shot. It might be more likely that a child would feign wellness and try to hide a symptom rather than risk peer attention, miss a social function, or get stuck with a needle. In all events, although mimicking is a possible cause of FEHL, support is flimsy at best. Moreover, a child who does mimic in this way may have unmet needs.

Getting Attention

All children seek attention and find ways to get it. "Getting attention" may have validity as a cause of FEHL, depending on how it is meant. If the FEHL is dismissively attributed to minor misbehavior, or to being manipulative, defiant, and so on ("you know how kids are"), then this author is highly skeptical. If, however, the implication is that the attention-seeking behavior is out of the ordinary or a possible sign of trouble, then this author agrees completely with this possibility. Displaying a false disorder, generally speaking, is not an emotionally healthy way to obtain attention. More to the point, ascribing FEHL to wanting attention might prevent considering a different underlying cause.

Illustrative Cases

Case 1

DT was a 9-year-old female referred because of failing a hearing screening at a health clinic. The mother and teacher noticed her hearing loss for 3 weeks. DT was considered learning disabled, and she had a marked seizure disorder that was not well controlled. She was not prone to ear problems. DT did not like school, perhaps because of the ridicule for her seizures, according to her mother. She said that DT felt bad about herself and described her as withdrawn and a poor eater who fought constantly. During the evaluation, DT was pleasant but did not respond to tones below 40 dB. Suspecting invalid performance, SRTs were sought and were found to be 5 dB. Returning to pure-tone audiometry, subtle hand movements and "no" headshakes on stimulus presentations were accepted as responses, and she passed a screening at 15 dB in each for tones 500 to 4000 Hz. She persisted in claiming that she did not hear well. The PSC score was very high at 53. After discussion, the mother realized that DT had emotional problems and accepted the recommendation of seeking mental health evaluation.

Case 2

LY, a 10-year-old female, failed a school hearing screening. Her schoolteachers had reported that the child did not pay attention to directions. The mother was not surprised because LY often failed to respond, had TV loud, and asked "what" more than others. She had minimal ENT trouble. She had done well in third grade the year before but only had Cs in fourth grade this past year. At the start of the evaluation, LY did not respond to most tones in her left ear up to 30 to 40 dB and not to any in her right ear up to 50 dB. The results were dubious, so SRTs were sought instead. The right SRT was 35 dB, supporting the notion of invalidity. Eventually, SRTs were 5 dB in each ear. Returning to pure-tone testing, responses gradually came at ever low levels to about 20 dB, but there were still many false negative responses. Word recognition scores at 30 dB HL were 80% in each ear, supporting the impression of little or no hearing loss. In the post-test discussion with the mother, it was learned that the parents divorced the year previous (just before the distinct drop in school performance). The girl missed her father and used to ask about him often, even though they saw each other regularly. She was described as "down on herself." The Pediatric Symptom Checklist score was positive at 30. Looking at the whole picture, the mother concluded that her daughter was distressed and she planned to seek mental health intervention for her.

Note that, in these cases, it was a hearing screening that led to contact with an audiologist, which in turn was the start of directing attention to psychosocial issues, echoing the quotation at the head of this chapter. Probably, even a nonexpert would suspect that these children were troubled. Finally, these cases also show the helpfulness of the Pediatric Symptom Checklist in supporting the clinician's suspicion of significant psychosocial disturbances.

Summary

The information in this chapter paints a rather gloomy picture of childhood FEHL. The reports do not say that children with FEHL are more or less like other kids, except for the false hearing loss. Instead, the evidence argues forcefully against the notion that children with FEHL are emotionally healthy but cunning deceivers seeking some palpable gain. False disorders can be considered "'body language,' a plea for help in a child who has no alternative method for communicating stress" and one that should not be taken lightly (Maisami & Freeman, 1987, p. 46).

Among children with FEHL, the hearing loss typically presented is moderate, bilateral, and sensorineural in essentially flat configuration. Most of the hearing losses fall between 40 and 60 dB, although the range is much wider. FEHL is twice as common in girls as in boys. The average age is 11 years with the majority of children in the range of 8 to 13 years.

The first concern about hearing usually arises from a failed hearing screening. The "hearing loss" comes on fairly rapidly of no obvious medical cause. In the clinic, most children follow normal conversation easily, which is frequently the tip-off that the hearing loss is not real.

The foremost cause of FEHL in children is some problem in life. Conflict at home or school is the rule. The children generally have a poor self-concept and feelings of insecurity, hostility, and aggression. Usually, these children are not performing at grade level, even though they are of normal intelligence or close to it. Often, the onset of the FEHL closely follows some specific, disturbing event, suggesting a causal link. False hearing loss can serve as protection in a frightening uncertain world. Delay in discovering FEHL increases the chance of its persistence, results in overlooking any psychosocial problems, and can result in inappropriate management. The next chapter explores the signs and risk factors of FEHL to help identify it as soon as possible.

Chapter 5

SIGNS AND RISK FACTORS

The mainstay of diagnosis is a lack of consistency in audiological testing.

—Pracy et al., 1996, p. 143

Introduction

Several signs and risk factors are red flags for invalid responding. Some are distinctly pretest factors, such as reason for referral; others are distinctly during-test factors, such as poor agreement between tone and speech thresholds. However, several of the behavioral signs do not fall neatly into either category and are common to both phases of the evaluation, such as straining to hear. Also, there is no clear distinction between factors that apply to adults versus children, except for obvious ones that are age related (e.g., schoolwork).

A caveat is that many of these signs and factors are seen in people who are doing their best during the evaluation. Distinguishing between invalid responders and genuine but struggling responders is a particularly apt example of the blending of the art and science of audiology. As clinicians gain experience, they develop a "feel" for the legitimacy of claims and behaviors. Yet, we must be wary of our clinical judgments and biases because there is a risk that our suspicions or "gut feelings" are wrong. Also, we need to guard against attributing too much significance to red-flag behaviors. We must not jump to conclusions. If a person has a genuine organic hearing impairment, it is a disservice to cast doubt on that disability without ample justification. A balance must be struck between being alert to clues and not being overly mistrustful.

Signs and Risk Factors Before Testing

There are four major categories of pretest clues for FEHL: (1) referral source, (2) reason for visit, (3) history, and (4) behavior.

Referral Source

Attorney

Referral by a lawyer means there is a legal question, one often involving compensation for a hearing loss alleged to stem from an illness, injury, or some source of liability.

Reason for Visit

Litigation

A patient may be referred by someone other than an attorney or be self-referred regarding a question of compensation through legal process, but it might not be at all evident at the outset. As part of any good evaluation, one of the first, if not the very first, questions is, "What brings you here?" or some similar query as to the goal of the assessment. At times, unless otherwise clear, the clinician might need to ask whether there is any legal action or potential legal action involved.

Financial Benefit

In addition to the above, there could be a strong monetary interest when an entitlement benefit is involved. Agencies might seek evaluation to determine eligibility or need for services and necessary devices.

Undesired Duty

A person may desire to avoid an objectionable duty (historically, military service), disagreeable responsibility, or unpleasant employment.

History

Many of the above items and a number of the ones that follow are not necessarily volunteered by the patient or patient's family. Some may need to be asked about. It is safe to say that the power of history-taking is underrated as a diagnostic tool.

Believability

One should be suspicious if the report of onset of the problem is strangely vague or if it is described as sudden (Jerger & Jerger, 1981) or rapidly developing but without an accompanying event. Most permanent hearing losses do not come on, whether in minutes or days, in isolation but have some related situation, such as an injury, illness, or identifiable syndrome, especially if bilateral. A report of a new, rapidly appearing hearing loss, particularly in children, with no logical cause must put us on the lookout for invalid test results. A truly sudden onset, particularly without discernible cause, is extremely rare in children (Psarommatis et al., 2009). A claim of a unilateral hearing impairment from being in an industrial setting is suspicious (Snyder, 2001), unless there had been one or a few exposures to a strong, blast-like sound on the "bad" side. Even then, one should expect at least some hearing loss in the opposite ear. Another way to look at the history is to ask oneself, does it make sense?

The following cases illustrate the point (Wang, Wang, Lin, & Lee, 2006). In unrelated incidences, two young women developed sudden bilateral hearing losses of no apparent physical cause. After an initial impression of genuine impairment, it was discovered that hearing was normal. Both women acknowledged enormous strain due to university entrance examinations; one was fearful of "hearing of failure."

In another example of an atypical history, a professional musician complained of a hearing loss in her left ear that began suddenly from no apparent cause (Monsell & Herzon, 1984). She had a similar episode in her right ear 8 years before with no recovery. Her audiologic results, obtained with good intratest and intertest reliability, showed the severe loss in the right ear and a moderate flat loss in the left ear. After a day of treatment, ABR testing was performed; it confirmed the severe loss in the right ear but indicated normal hearing in the left ear. It was then learned through psychiatric intervention that the patient was under terrible stress related to career and marital conflicts. She "couldn't bear to hear" things her husband said to her. Consistent with a conversion reaction, she had a dependent, pathologic, marital relationship with a domineering father figure, which appeared symbolically as a hearing impairment to avoid hearing the unacceptable things he said. Although this is an example of obtaining a dubious history, it might also be an example of obtaining an incomplete history. A suspicious report should prompt further probing. Had the information about her unfortunate situation been elicited at the initial interview, the case might have been viewed differently. In instances of sudden hearing losses or any loss whose onset is out of the ordinary, one should ask not only about physical events but also about disturbing events.

School Problems

Probably the most common report about children with FEHL is a school problem in the past year, mainly a drop in grades but also poor conduct, social conflicts, or wanting to stay home. Regardless of the cause, many such children are troubled and are more likely to present unreliable and invalid test results.

New Uncharacteristic Behaviors

A change in behavioral patterns, without a satisfactory explanation, should put the clinician on guard. Examples are moodiness, less interest in a hobby, eating significantly less or more, and hypo- or hypersomnia. Among other signs in children are gloominess, acting less mature, and spending more time alone.

Abuse

As seen previously, abuse can underlie a false hearing loss in children. Sometimes information from outside or from the informant might allude to some abuse. If not, but the clinician forms a suspicion, it may be worth exploring that possibility. There is further discussion of maltreatment in Chapter 10, Psychosocial Considerations, and of ways to bring up and probe sensitive issues in Chapter 11, Management.

Observations and Behavior

Children who portray a false hearing loss converse remarkably well without visual clues when they do not feel they are being tested.

Patients who present false hearing loss may have a normal social style but some may exhibit patterns out of the ordinary. They can act passive, anxious, or ingratiating (Jerger & Jerger, 1981). Yet, some patients also are overly animated or hostile. Some are quite upset by their hearing loss; others show a surprising nonchalance, an abnormal lack of concern called *la belle indifférence* (Wolf, Birger, Ben-Shoshan, & Kronenberg, 1993). Children and youth might seem argumentative and contrary, but are more likely to present a sullen, subdued manner or a flat affect.

Patients have been noted to give remarkable and excessive detail about the onset and cause of their hearing impairment (Rintelmann & Schwan, 1999). They may volunteer information not asked about (Martin, 2009). They are more likely to overstate the distress bought about by the hearing loss. Keep in mind, however, that a person who has experienced a frightening episode can be highly sensitized to the event and feel the need to recount it in great detail.

If a patient reports years of severe bilateral hearing loss, but speech as well as vocal pitch and loudness are normal, the clinician must be wary. Patients may claim very good lip-reading skills to explain how well he or she seems to understand yet continue to follow a conversation even when they cannot see the speaker's mouth. Patients might go through "excessive contortions" (Rintelmann & Schwan, 1999) to watch faces, cup a hand over an ear, lean toward the speaker, and strain excessively to hear. A person wearing a hearing aid might adjust it frequently, claim extraordinary benefit from amplification, profess routine use but be unfamiliar with the instrument, or give implausible estimates of battery cost and life.

Types of Nontest Inconsistencies

The chapter's opening sentiment that the mainstay of diagnosis is a lack of consistency in audiologic testing is heartily agreed with. However, that truism might unintentionally divert attention from the nontest inconsistencies. Diagnosis includes not only tests but also case history and observations. Understandably, clinicians rely on the array of very good tests, but one may wonder if that fosters an underreliance on observations and history.

Many ailments are diagnosed on the basis of observed behaviors and reported symptoms and are not easily verified by laboratory tests. A diagnosis that leans heavily on history and observations is strongly influenced by the extent to which the clinician believes the patient and thus regards a complaint as an illness, not a deception. Necessarily, the factor most relied on must be consistency. Multiple sources of information can be compared and, therefore, can form the basis of inconsistencies. They include inconsistency: within the history, between history and observed behavior, in history obtained from the patient versus history from an informant, between the patient's history and medical records, among different examinations over time, and between history and other sources of information about the patient (Sharpe, 2003). However, bear in mind that even some nonlitigants will show a degree of inconsistency in symptom presentation, particularly if distressed (Main, 2003).

Signs During Testing

The signs of FEHL during the actual testing consist of behaviors and audiometric indicators. Again, there is the caution that some of these behavioral and audiometric signs are seen in people who are participating in the evaluation to the best of their ability.

Pure-Tone Audiometry

Behaviors

Logically, some of the pretest behaviors that raise suspicion continue into the testing phase, such as understanding soft speech when the patient cannot see the speaker's mouth and straining to hear. In the test booth, a patient may concentrate strenuously to prove cooperation, or act bored, look around the test room, adjust clothing, and the like. Other behaviors are frequent comments about being confused or having ringing in ears, facial expressions of being uncertain or confused, and radiating the impression of being quite cooperative (McCanna & DeLapa, 1981). One trick some informed patients use is self-masking by humming or teeth grinding, thereby raising their own thresholds (Gaynor, 1974). Clinicians can listen for self-generated sounds via the audiometer's talk-back circuit.

Note the subjective nature of many of the above descriptors, such as, appears to be straining, looking confused. Often, the judgment is a matter of whether those behaviors seem merely more pronounced than usual as opposed to being genuinely excessive, keeping in mind that people have widely varying personalities and styles. The clinician must decide when a difference in degree becomes a difference in kind, that is, whether the behavior deviates sufficiently from the norm to be suspicious for FEHL.

Reliability

The foremost audiometric sign in pure-tone audiometry is lack of reliability. By and large, in clinical testing, thresholds on repeated measures fall within 5 dB. There is general agreement that discrepancies should not be more than 10 dB at any frequency, and if they are, one must consider the possibility of FEHL. Another sort of poor agreement, albeit infrequent, is bone-conduction results that are worse than air conduction results by 10 dB or more. By random variations, bone-conduction thresholds may be slightly poorer than air-conduction thresholds (Martin & Clark, 2009). A consistent pattern of bone conduction worse than air by 10 dB or more at several frequencies requires the audiologist to check for some artifact; if none, one should consider this a sign of invalid performance that needs resolution.

One school of thought is that there is a continuum of consistency from high to low corresponding to conversion disorder and to malingering. The idea is that patients with a conversion disorder, because of their conviction that they are hearing impaired, are more consistent than malingering patients (Austen & Lynch, 2004). A case in point is the musician mentioned above with the unlikely history of a sudden loss in each ear separated by years, who had good intratest and intertest reliability and eventually was considered to have a conversion disorder. In contrast, Snyder (2001), although agreeing that conscious intention varies greatly, feels that all audiometric and audiologic clues for false hearing loss are the same regardless of the degree of intentionality. There is not a consensus on this question of consistency and intentionality. Some invalid responders may be consistent, even on repeated testing. Perhaps, they lie more at the conversion disorder end. In all events, it is safest to say that a lack of reliability strongly suggests FEHL, but good reliability is no guarantee that results are valid.

"Plus or Minus" (± dB) and "Within." Agreement between audiologic measures of sensitivity often is described in two ways: "plus or minus" and "within." It may seem self-understood or trivial, but it is worth pointing out that they are not equivalent. "Plus or minus 5" (±5 dB) means that a minimum response level could vary from 5 dB higher to 5 dB lower than some tentative threshold and thereby encompass a range of 10 dB. In contrast, "within 5" means precisely that, a range not exceeding 5 dB. To illustrate, if a tentative hearing threshold is 55 dB, ±5 dB means (or at least could be construed to mean) that sometimes there are no responses until 60 dB (+5) and, at other times, there are apparently credible responses at 50 dB (–5). Most likely, many clinicians would consider a 10-dB response range, such as this, as stretching the limit of good reliability. If, however, a person never responds at 50 dB, responds about half the time at 55 dB, and always responds at 60 dB, that would be deemed good reliability. The same holds true if the person always responds at 55 dB and occasionally responds at 50 dB but never lower. In either case, the response range is within 5 dB and is probably more typical of a good responder.

False Negative and False Positive Responses

A false negative response is failing to respond to a perceptible signal. A false positive response is responding when there is no perceptible signal, either because no signal is presented or because it is below the true threshold. By definition, persons with FEHL have more false negative responses than normal responders. They also make many fewer false positive responses than do true responders. Chaiklin and Ventry (1965) analyzed false positive rates in patients with FEHL. In one portion of the study, sampling periods of 60 seconds of silence were interspersed during regular audiometry. False positive responses occurred in 55% of non-FEHL subjects and in 10% of FEHL patients, even though the investigators expressly fostered false positive responses by encouraging subjects to respond even when they were *uncertain* if they had heard a tone. Rates of false positive responses any time during the audiometry were 86% for those with true hearing loss and 22% for those in the FEHL group. Incidentally, if patients were likely to give false positive responses, they were about as likely to do so in the first 30 seconds as in the second 30 seconds.

When a test signal is strong enough, it can be felt even though not heard. Generally speaking, signals from a bone-conduction transducer become tactually perceptible with mastoid placement at 30 dB for 250 Hz, and 55 dB for 500 Hz (Goodhill, 1979; Nober, 1970). By air conduction through supra-aural earphones, signals are perceptible at 75 dB for 125 Hz, 90 dB for 250 Hz, and 100 dB at 500 Hz. Failure to respond at levels known to be tactually perceptible is quite likely a false negative response, although using such high signals is seldom needed.

Manner

The quality of response can be revealing, that is, its briskness, timing, and clarity. Very slight finger or hand movements time-locked to a stimulus can be telltale. Is the patient's manner slow, elaborate, deliberate, or laborious? Green (1978), in an entertaining way, reported UFO sightings, that is, "useful finger observations," in assessing the quality of a response. He described various finger responses and their likely significance. Two were associated with feigning. The first was a delayed reaction after a tone was on longer than usual, which he dubbed the "malingafinger." The other was, as a droll parallel to escalating inflationary values, the "inflation index" finger, that is, the minimum response level gets higher and higher. To illustrate, suppose in an ascending technique that the first response comes at 30 dB HL. Upon a second ascending approach, the patient fails to response until 35 dB HL is reached, and yet another ascending run does not elicit a response until 40 dB. The opposite, is the "fallsalarm finger" (a.k.a., the "reverse malingafinger"), referring to excessive false positive responses. The "fallsalarm finger" responders generally are overeager in trying to present genuine thresholds or they may have tinnitus. Although frustrating and adding difficulty to the test, Green felt that the "fallsalarm finger" is highly unlikely among persons with FEHL.

Configuration

The most common audiometric configurations in false hearing loss are flat and saucer shaped (sometimes also called trough-shaped or, colloquially, "cookie bite"), but there is considerable variability. For example, in reporting on 39 school children with FEHL, Yoshida, Noguchi, and Uemura (1989) found that one third did not have flat or saucer-shaped configurations but instead displayed a variety of contours. Similarly, in their classic study of 64 veterans with FEHL, Ventry and Chaiklin (1965b) found only 8% with saucer-shaped patterns; moreover, saucer-shaped patterns also were seen in some of their organic hearing loss group.

A configuration in false hearing loss may resemble equal loudness contours but that is when hearing is normal. However, the clinician usually would not know ahead of time whether the patient has some degree of organic loss. Probably the reason that only 8% of Ventry and Chaiklin's (1965b) patients had saucer-shaped patterns was because, as military veterans, many also had an organic component, which would alter an otherwise saucer shape. Even then, the configurations of their FEHL group may represent, to some extent, equal loudness patterns but not necessarily in a saucer shape (Ventry & Chaiklin, 1965b). To explain, if a hearing loss is exaggerated, the configurations of the true and the false loss are combined. Also, overlays tend to produce a "flatter" or more gently sloping audiogram than would have been found otherwise (Snyder, 2001). If there is a cochlear high-frequency loss or a notch pattern, recruitment tends to flatten an exaggerated presentation (Coles,

2001). The reason is that equal loudness contours become flatter with increasing intensity (Gelfand, 1998). Finally, it is paramount to bear in mind that flat or saucer patterns appear in persons with true losses, and saucer-shaped configurations have been linked to some congenital, genetic conditions.

Looking at the matter from the other side, a steep high-frequency loss or a notch configuration is evidence of genuine organic hearing loss. Such patterns are virtually unheard of in false hearing loss. Patients are not sophisticated enough to produce a hearing loss only in a certain frequency range. Almost always, 4000- to 6000-Hz notch patterns are caused by excessive sound level exposure. Conversely, damage from high sound level is almost entirely confined to high frequencies (excepting blast acoustic trauma, which can cause a hearing loss across frequencies from damage to the cochlea or to the conductive mechanism). Thus, in claims of hearing loss from high noise exposure, a loss at 500 Hz exceeding 25 dB HL should raise suspicion (Coles, 2001). Rickards, deVidi, and McMahon (1996) found that, in a group with a history of high-level noise exposure, 93% of reliable responders had 500-Hz thresholds at 20 dB HL or better, whereas 94% of unreliable responders had thresholds worse than 20 dB (see Snyder, 2001 for more details). But, with regard to FEHL, pure-tone patterns are too variable to have any diagnostic significance.

Lack of Crossover

In severe unilateral losses, the lack of a crossover response when the opposite ear is not masked is highly indicative of a false hearing loss. Depending on frequency, the usual interaural attention for air conduction with supra-aural earphones is about 60 dB. Thus, even a person with no hearing in one ear and normal hearing in the other ear would produce an audiogram for the bad ear in the vicinity of 60 dB HL due to cross-hearing. Once interaural attention levels are exceeded, a shadow curve emerges that mirrors the configuration of hearing in the better ear. However, interaural attenuation covers a range of 40 to 70 dB, depending on frequency and subject. Because in individual cases we cannot know what the interaural attenuation is, it becomes problematic whether the lack of responses at 70 dB HL indicates invalid behavior. Certainly, there should be a response by 80 dB due to crossover (Snyder, 1973). Insert tube earphones add, conservatively, 15 dB of interaural attention, such that lack of a crossover response would be ambiguous up to 95 dB HL (making supra-aural earphones preferable in cases of suspected FEHL). Bone-conduction (BC) testing has the advantage, in this context, of hardly any interaural attention, perhaps 0 to 5 dB. Thus, a patient should respond to bone-conduction signals near the threshold levels of the better ear, regardless of which side the bone-conduction transducer is placed on. Failure to respond when the transducer is on the poor side almost surely is a false negative.

Maxwell and Brooks (1986) reported an apt example. A man presented a 45-dB unilateral hearing loss with only a minor, 8-dB air-bone gap while the good ear was not masked. The patient acknowledged a great deal of stress, which later resolved, and then his audiograms were normal in the next 2 years.

This author had a striking example of absent bone-conduction responses in a dubious unilateral hearing loss. With the tone on, the examiner moved a bone-conduction oscillator in steps from the mastoid of the good ear over the head to the mastoid of the "impaired" ear. The boy readily acknowledged perception when the oscillator was on the mastoid on the good side. As oscillator placement approached the vertex, he reported decreasing loudness; after crossing the top of the head to the "bad" side, he reported only faint sound until the signal was denied entirely when the mastoid of the "bad ear" eventually was reached. The examiner varied the oscillator location, and the magnitude of admitted loudness systematically corresponded to the distance from the mastoid of the "bad" ear.

Speech Audiometry

Pure-Tone and Speech Threshold Agreement

The primary value of measuring a speech recognition threshold is the cross-validation of tone thresholds. The pure-tone average (PTA), whether the Carhart three-frequency average of 500, 1000, and 2000 Hz or the Fletcher average of the two best thresholds of those frequencies, if the configuration is other than fairly flat, should agree with the SRT within about 6 dB. Lack of agreement between tone and speech thresholds is a hallmark of FEHL, invariably with the speech threshold lower than the PTA. However, comparing speech and tone thresholds supposes not only that the tone thresholds are reliable, but that the speech threshold is too. As with tones, intratest reliability for speech should be within 5 dB and no more than 10 dB.

An SRT that is lower than the PTA by 12 dB or more is a prime indicator of FEHL (Rintelmann & Schwan, 1999; Snyder, 2001). When there is a difference between the two, the consensus is that the speech threshold is much closer to the genuine threshold. Even if the tone thresholds and the speech threshold are tenuous but the regions of uncertainty are separated, one has a trustworthy indicator of false results. For example, if tone "thresholds" are in a range of 40 to 55 dB HL and the speech "threshold" is in a range of 20 to 35 dB HL, there is a definite difference, which is diagnostic of invalid results.

Loudness Perception

The reason for the PTA-SRT difference favoring the SRT is not entirely clear but must involve the sense of loudness of different sounds. Ventry (1976b) offered this explanation. Evidence had shown that, at suprathreshold levels, people judged spondees and pure tones to be equally loud at the same SPL, but audiometers are calibrated in Hearing Level (HL). For 1000 Hz, the SPL reference is 7 dB SPL, and for speech recognition, the reference is 20 dB SPL.[1] A false hearing loss of 60 dB at 1000 Hz converts to 67 dB SPL (60 + 7). A person using a loudness yardstick consistently would present an SRT of 45 dB HL, which converts to 65 dB SPL (45 + 20). Thus, the two signals have nearly identical SPLs but much different HLs with the SRT appearing inordinately low. The 15-dB difference coincides with the Ventry and Chaiklin (1965a) study in which the majority of subjects had a speech-tone difference of at least 13 dB. Although using

---

[1]The exact values depend on the particular earphone but these values are within 0.5 dB and suitable for our purposes.

some logic, this hypothesis has its limitations (Martin, 2009). For one thing, it seems at odds with the different loudnesses of broadband and narrowband signals at the same overall intensity level.

There are two main factors in the difference in loudness between speech and tones at the same amplitude. First is bandwidth. A broadband signal is louder than a narrowband signal at the same level, because loudness summates as the number of critical bands increases (Gelfand, 1998). Speech is a broadband sound, whereas pure tones are the narrowest of sounds. The second factor is the rate of loudness growth for different frequencies. As intensity increases, loudness growth is steeper for low frequencies than for high frequencies. A look at a minimum audibility curve shows that at a low level, say 20 dB SPL, frequencies below about 200 Hz are inaudible, but at a moderate level of 70 dB SPL, frequency audibility extends down to about 50 Hz. Similarly, equal loudness contours illustrate that, at low sound pressure level, tones equal the loudness of a 1000-Hz tone down to 400 Hz. But, at a moderate level the contour of equal loudness extends lower to about 170 Hz. As a result, raising the signal from very low to a moderate intensity not only makes more low frequencies audible but it also increases the loudness of the low frequencies more than the loudness of any other tonal region. We can experience this ourselves by listening to music at a comfortable level and then turning the volume down. One notes an absence of the bass region. Turning the volume way up brings out proportionately more bass (Gelfand, 1998).

Unusual Behavior During Speech Audiometry

There are red flag behaviors and responses, which are out of the ordinary, seem suspicious, or defy logic. Some apply just to the SRT, but most apply to both the SRT and suprathreshold word recognition scoring.

- Half word response during SRT (e.g., "ear" for "eardrum." seen almost exclusively in false responders)
- Repeat one syllable of a spondee a few times (as if struggling to respond)

- Nonsensical errors of just one sound (e.g., "ridewalk" for "sidewalk")
- Sudden stopping or starting of correct responses
- Averting the eyes or a slight head turn toward the side of the ear being stimulated but no oral response
- Protesting, "I can't hear you. You're too soft," but otherwise responding to offhand remarks at or below the speech threshold
- Pressing the earphone to the ear
- Bizarre response or error by association: "dig" for "ditch," "boxcar" for "railroad"
- Rising inflection, as if a question or a guess: "pick?" "sidewalk?"
- Delayed response after a few seconds
- Rhyming responses, even if nonsense syllables
- Seemingly deliberate errors
- Exaggerated straining to understand during the test.

Physiologic Measures

Otoacoustic Emissions

If otoacoustic emissions (OAE) are clearly present, a supposed hearing loss greater than 40 dB would be highly suspicious for the frequencies where OAEs were found (Hall, 2000).

Acoustic Reflex Threshold (ART)

An ART of 10 dB or less above voluntary auditory threshold is so low as to be a sign that the voluntary threshold is inflated (Gelfand, Schwander, & Silman, 1990). Logically, an AR below a voluntary threshold indicates an invalid auditory threshold.

Summary

Prominent risk factors for FEHL include a question of litigation, an atypical history, and exaggerated patient attempts to display communicative difficulty, such as straining to hear.

Often, the first audiometric sign of FEHL is response inconsistency. The single best indicator of FEHL is finding speech thresholds better than tone thresholds by 10 dB or more. Other suggestive behaviors are slow or elaborate responses, absence of a shadow curve in severe unilateral cases, protests of, "I can't hear it," responses to soft offhand remarks, and pressing the earphone against the ear.

During speech audiometry, noteworthy markers are half-word responses to spondees, a rising quizzical inflection, and a high responding to informal speech at a low sensation level. Finally, if there is a supposed hearing loss of 45 dB or more, but OAEs are normal or the ART is 10 dB or less above volunteered threshold, one has virtual certainty that voluntary responses are invalid. The task then is to resolve the questions of validity and obtain an accurate measurement of the person's hearing. The next three chapters discuss ways to do just that.

Chapter 6

CONVENTIONAL BEHAVIORAL AUDIOMETRY

One of the most interesting and yet challenging tasks the audiologist is called upon to perform is the identification and evaluation of functional or nonorganic hearing loss.

—Kinstler, Phelan, and Lavender, 1972, p. 187

Introduction

Chapter 5 enumerated the many factors that might signal invalid test performance. This chapter looks at ways to assess hearing using conventional behavioral tests and their modifications. Chapter 7 also addresses behavioral procedures but those designed specially for FEHL.

Behavioral audiometry involves patient participation, specifically, some intentional physical reaction to sound. In contrast, objective procedures bypass patient participation, and require only passive cooperation while an instrument directly measures and records some involuntary physiologic reaction to sound. There are a few other ways to categorize auditory tests. They can be grouped according to whether they are qualifying versus quantifying, that is, whether they merely identify invalid results or provide an estimate of genuine auditory thresholds, which is more difficult. However, this division may be less meaningful because the distinction between qualitative and quantitative is not always hard and fast. Sometimes electrophysiologic procedures have been called direct tests because, like objective and quantifying approaches, they are independent of a patient's performance. Direct procedures do measure some aspect of auditory function directly, but they are not direct tests of hearing. Clinicians prefer one term over another, but the essential distinction is between behavioral and nonbehavioral tests.

Setting the Stage

When it comes to FEHL, behavioral tests should not be thought of as less valuable than electrophysiologic tests. To the contrary, they often are preferable and more efficient. Objective tests can be extremely helpful but might not be necessary if standard approaches and their modifications are used effectively (Nilo & Saunders, 1976; Snyder, 2001). Behavioral tests also have the advantages of simplicity and convenience (Hosoi, Tsuta, Murata, & Levitt, 1999; Pracy et al., 1996) without the considerable cost of electrophysiologic procedures.

Performing behavioral audiometry is deceptively easy. In other words, it is harder than it looks, especially when done well. Nowhere is this more true than in the case of patients who do not respond in a typical fashion or whose results seem at odds with pretest hearing behavior. The audiologist's desire (or pressure in some settings) to complete all the standard tests, and to do so quickly, reduces the vigilance and astuteness to spot an invalid responder.

Before testing is begun, audiologists should have formed an idea of a patient's hearing ability. With practice, one can estimate whether a person has little or no hearing loss, some loss, or a great deal of hearing loss. This is a good routine to follow with all patients.

Facility with Equipment

Success in evaluating patients with questionable results requires blending knowledge and technical facility. All procedures must be conducted with confidence, and going from one test to another should be seamless. Smooth, efficient audiometric technique is as important as the tests, themselves. It is essential, therefore, that the clinician be highly familiar with the equipment and its capabilities. Equipment manuals should be read thoroughly and procedures should be practiced on real, or even imaginary, subjects in order to perform all procedures well and shift among them quickly. Working with patients who do not respond validly demands more concentration than usual. This can be accomplished best when not having to think about which buttons to push or which key to press.

Sources of Inconsistencies

Test inconsistencies have three sources: equipment, tester, and patient (Engelberg, 1970). Regarding the "hardware," if results are highly unusual, one must follow the first rule of audiometry and ensure that, indeed, the equipment is turned on. Check power cords and cables. An intermittent signal due to a broken earphone cord can play havoc with reliability. Make sure that the earphones are on the proper ear, that the pinna is not folded over the ear canal opening, and that the canal does not collapse from the earphone pressing on the pinna. The most typical culprit is controls that are not set correctly. A good example of an incorrect setting is when there is no response while testing a particular ear. If truthful, most audiologists, including this writer, will confess to having had the transducer selector erroneously on "bone" rather than on "right" or "left" or to similar errors.

Another factor to consider when results are dubious is the patient's status. Check if the person is not feeling well, in pain, very tired, upset, and so forth (Coles, 2001). Maybe the patient just needs reinstruction regarding attention and the proper response.

Perhaps less evident is that the clinician may be the source of the problem. It is remarkably easy, even for veteran clinicians, to move one's head or eyes up and down in sync with tone presentations or to produce hand and body cues in conducting and scoring various tests. Also, we must guard against the tendency to fall into a rhythmic pattern when presenting pure tones. Finally, clinicians are not immune to presupposing, jumping to conclusions, or expecting (erroneously) to find some particular results.

Audiologist's Emotions

The challenge and frustrations encountered with FEHL cases can provoke an array of emotions (Engelberg, 1970). The process of evaluating an unreliable responder is often aggravating and emotionally tiring. The clinician needs to be vigilant about feelings of indignation, dislike for the patient, and so forth. Also, when we detect a FEHL or "nail" a true threshold, we must guard against feelings of exuberance or victory. Other sentiments that we are vulnerable to are embarrassment at admitting that we cannot obtain valid results or the temptation to "put something down" on paper despite great uncertainty to safeguard our image

A standard recommendation is that clinicians should not be judgmental when they think someone is being deceitful. On the other hand, it is important to remember that clinicians are human, too. Naturally, they might feel resentful when treated dishonestly, especially because they see themselves in a helping role. Clinicians need to accept their own natural inclinations toward indignation or irritation, recognize them as extraclinical, and bear in mind the overriding obligation to perform their duties with professionalism.

Rintelmann and Schwan (1999) cautioned that evaluating FEHL is not a game of "matching wits" with the patient. Although that is true, the reality is that at times the clinician and the patient may be trying to figure out what the other is doing to achieve their particular goals. This writer prefers an alternative characterization: using techniques, which might include some cat-and-mouse matching of wits, not as an adversary, but as an astute clinician.

Patient Strategies and Sophistication

We probably could make it harder for a person to present a false hearing loss or an exaggeration, if we knew how patients went about invalidating audiologic tests. They likely employ different tactics, some depending on their state of mind (such as a conversion disorder or malingering), and others depending on their imagination and personality. We cannot simply ask patients how they do it for the self-evident reason that patients are striving to mislead (Martin, 2009).

Martin, Champlin, and McCreery (2001) resorted to asking normal-hearing adults to feign hearing loss, motivated them by paying them according to how well they feigned, and then asked them to describe the strategies they used. Most subjects said that at first they responded haphazardly but then they used an internal loudness criterion to decide when to respond at different frequencies or during retesting. After being tested for a while, subjects realized that a set procedure was being used. In order to be consistent, they began counting the number of tones in a sequence. Because actual patients with FEHL might adopt such a strategy, it would be wise to deviate from a fixed technique and present tones at random intensities.

Third Parties Observing

When a patient showed evidence of better hearing than supposed, this clinician found it very beneficial to have an accompanying person observe. For privacy and legal reasons, there should be a justification for the escorting person to observe the testing, for example, being a partner or relative or a child's parents/guardians. If a person can witness the better hearing, he or she is far more likely to believe the clinician's assessment. This must be arranged unobtrusively, and in the case of adults, with the patient's permission. The clinician can tell the adult patient that the partner might like to watch the testing and ask if there is an objection. The clinician also needs to contrive a situation to have the partner/parent join. The other party should be informed ahead of time that you feel hearing is better than believed and you wanted to demonstrate it discreetly. The observer can be seated in the control booth and listen via the talkback monitor or they can be in the same room with the patient and clinician during conversation. The goal is to demonstrate the person's better hearing without the patient being aware of the motive. This requires tact and cleverness.

Pure-Tone Audiometry

Instructions

Precise instructions are essential with any patient but even more so when validity is in doubt. Misunderstanding can lead to low reliability, and one can minimize ambiguity by instructing well. Instruct the patient face to face rather than through earphones; earphones imply testing, and the patient may request a stronger signal. By complying, the audiologist inadvertently helps the patient establish a loudness standard (Snyder, 2001). Instructions must be simple, explicit, concise, and emphatic to respond as soon as the tone is heard, no matter how soft, and to stop responding as soon as the tone is gone (Engelberg, 1970; Snyder, 2001). Instructions should not be wordy or technical. Leave out extraneous tasks. All that one needs to do and should do is to specify the stimulus and the response: a tone and a hand raise (Engelberg, 1970).

A practice that this examiner finds helpful is to model the desired response by raising his hand while instructing to "raise your hand, even if you think you hear it." Clinicians may vary in their opinion as to whether the response should be raising a finger or a hand. Probably more important than what is moving is how clearly it is moving (i.e., if it is a definite, well-timed motion). If the patient becomes less consistent or responses more difficult to judge, the patient can be reminded through the talk-over circuit to respond clearly every time. As a rule, responses become more reliable and less ambiguous when the patient is merely told to make a crisper motion.

Some clinicians prefer a button-press over a hand-raising response because of ease and speed. As seen in Chapter 5, Signs and Risk Factors, observing a patient's response movements can be most useful. It is true that a button-press response can save time; for an air-conduction audiogram, test time is reduced by an average of one minute per ear (DiGiovanni & Repka, 2007). However, the qualitative aspects of responses are not available from pressing a button, because the response is all or nothing (Martin & Clark, 2009). The indicator light either comes on or it does not. The increased test speed may not outweigh the benefits of the behavioral observations. Very slight movements of the finger or hand—or for that matter of the face, eyes, head, and body—that are time-locked to a stimulus can be informative. This author feels that, in behavioral audiometry, clinicians should give greater weight to the benefits of observing behavior than a blinking light.

The patient's positioning is important. The patient should not face the examiner so as not to be able to watch the clinician. The clinician's routine and incidental movements can prompt false responses, even in an honest patient. The opposite, having the patient's back to the tester, prevents the tester from noticing subtle body language and facial gestures mentioned above. Seating a patient at 90 degrees to the tester is preferable even during routine audiometry (Martin & Clark, 2009), let alone when there is a patient who is not responding properly.

This recalls the case of a woman claiming a very severe hearing loss and wearing binaural body hearing aids. Her affect seemed vaguely unusual. Using low-level speech and warble tones in a sound field without her hearing aids, her eyes flicked slightly to the right or left according to which loudspeaker was presenting the signals. These localization behaviors were consistent at 20 dB HL.

Starting Levels

Virtually all authorities advocate that, as soon as suspicion of FEHL arises, whether before or during testing, one should proceed with very low signals in ascending fashion to avoid having the patient establish a loudness reference. If normal hearing is not found, one can check validity by comparing tone and/or speech thresholds obtained through ascending and descending runs. This approach is discussed later in this chapter. As a reliability check after several frequencies have been tested, retest the first frequency; if there is a discrepancy beyond 5 dB, consider verifying additional thresholds.

Small Steps

Another consideration is using small steps of 2 dB for speech and tones (Nilo & Saunders, 1976). As Snyder (2001) points out, a person hearing a series of tones at increasing intensity will eventually decide that the signal is loud enough for a response. Raising the signal in 5-dB steps would cover a larger span than raising it in 2-dB steps before obtaining a response. For example, if a person decided to respond by the fourth presentation, and the starting point was 30 dB HL, 2-dB increments would cover 6 dB (30, 32, 34, 36 dB) whereas 5-dB increments would cover 15 dB (30, 35, 40, 45 dB).

Tinnitus

Tinnitus might lead to false-positive responses and, thus, to inconsistency during pure-tone audiometry. One way to check for tinnitus is to use several seconds of silence between signals. Excessive false-positive responses may indicate either an overly scrupulous patient or tinnitus. An additional check is to ask the patient if they hear tinnitus during a silent period. Tell the person that there will be no signal presented for several seconds and to report when asked if any sound or ringing had been heard. If the person does not hear any sound, reiterate the above instructions to respond to soft sounds but only when fairly sure there was a sound. If the person does report having heard tinnitus, consider using warble tones, pulsed tones, or, less preferably, narrowband noises. Using a long interstimulus interval helps monitor patient accuracy.

Pulsed tones and warble tones can help the patient distinguish the test signal from the tinnitus. ASHA guidelines (American Speech-Language-Hearing Association, 2005) for pure-tone audiometry allow for pulsed and warble tones. Thresholds for continuous, pulsed, warbled, and pulsed-warble tones are more or less equivalent for normal hearers (Burk & Wiley, 2004; Dockum & Robinson, 1975; Franklin, Johnson, Smith-Olinde, & Nicholson, 2009). Mineau and Schlauch (1997) compared thresholds obtained using pulsed tones (200 ms on-off) and continuous tones (1–2 sec) in subjects with tonal tinnitus. Thresholds were nearly identical, test-retest reliability was equivalent, and there were fewer false positive responses during pulsed-tone testing.

Narrowband noises are another acceptable signal. Even though they are not calibrated for measuring auditory thresholds, they are calibrated for effective masking. Generally, the SPLs for narrowband masking noises are ±3 dB of the corresponding dB HL for pure tones (Wilbur, 2002). Thresholds for pure tones, warble tones, and narrowband noises are equally reliable and generally within 3 dB for persons with normal hearing (Orchik & Rintelmann, 1978). It may be better to get fairly reliable thresholds for narrowband noises than to get untrustworthy results for pure or warble tones. Regardless of stimulus, the clinician should reinforce with praise, not just correct responses, but also correct nonresponses during no-signal periods. For example, one could say, "That's right. You did not raise your hand in the previous several seconds, and I did not present a sound then." Conversely, the clinician can discourage false positives by nicely informing the person of the error, "No, I didn't make a sound that last time. I know it can be difficult but try to be sure you hear my sound."

If spending too much time on one frequency in one ear because of inconsistency, whether due to tinnitus or not, don't get stuck there. It may be better to test one tone with fair accuracy in each ear and then move on to other frequencies alternating between ears rather than laboriously testing 250 to 8000 Hz in one ear and wearing down tester and patient before switching to the other ear.

Speech Audiometry

A common recommendation is to begin with or switch to speech audiometry at the earliest inkling of FEHL. The basic principles for pure-tone audiometry apply to speech audiometry: effective instructing, low starting point with ascending technique, and small steps (Nilo & Saunders, 1976). If one has begun with pure-tone testing and wishes to switch, face-to-face instructions for speech audiometry may not be practical. However, if one starts the session with speech audiometry, face-to-face communication without earphones is preferable.

It may go without saying that, during speech audiometry, the patient must not be able to see the speaker's face, particularly a patient who might be presenting a false or exaggerated hearing loss. Once again, the 90-degree angle is advantageous. If the patient looks toward the clinician, the clinician should direct the patient to look straight ahead. Incidentally, if the clinician feels it necessary to block visual cues, one should not hold a hand or sheet of paper near the mouth, especially between the mouth and the microphone. These alter the sound spectrum arriving at the microphone. An alternative is a specially designed fabric screen that hides the mouth but is acoustically porous.

In obtaining a speech recognition threshold, familiarizing the patient with the spondaic words is recommended as a routine practice (Martin & Clark, 2009; Olsen & Matkin, 1991). It is even more valuable with FEHL in order to minimize ambiguity and to make the task more concrete. The audiologist can either have the person repeat the words (as a "practice" run) or give the patient a list of the words to read. Instructions must be explicit to repeat those words, even if very soft, and patients should be urged to guess when uncertain (Martin & Clark, 2009; Snyder, 2001). During testing, use a commanding but not overly demanding voice; it is counterproductive to antagonize. As soon as the patient repeats the spondee, give the next one promptly. Increase the rate of presentation. This encourages responding and gives no time to wonder whether or not to respond (Engelberg, 1970).

The recommended mode of presenting test words during speech audiometry, particularly for the word recognition score (WRS), is through recorded means. However, when dealing with FEHL, monitored live voice (MLV) has advantages. Dixon and Newby (1959) advised switching to monitored live voice at the first indication of FEHL. The clinician can manipulate the situation much better by MLV, such as encouraging, cajoling, and interspersing informal remarks to obtain more valid responses. Moreover, the patient reaction to "live voice provides the diagnostician with many delicate, useful clues which might well be lost if the stimuli were . . . recorded" (Kintsler, Phelan, & Lavender, 1972, p. 190).

To achieve a high WRS, normal hearers need a minimum signal of about 27 dB above the SRT (see Olsen & Matkin, 1991). Thus, one tactic to check for FEHL is to give the test words at a low sensation level of 10 dB. If the person achieves a WRS of 94 to 100%, then the SRT must be exaggerated. The actual sensation level must be at least 15 dB higher than the supposed 10 dB SL to approach the 27 dB SL needed to achieve such a high score. This information can help to estimate the true SRT. Suppose that a person's voluntary SRT was 35 dB HL and the WRS was 92% at 10 dB SL. Reasoning backward, as the true SRT must be 15 dB better than the voluntary SRT, then the true SRT cannot be worse than 20 dB HL. On the other hand, if at 10 dB SL the WRS is below 94%, one should readminister the test and add 15 dB SL; the score should rise substantially in conductive and most cochlear impairments.

Managing Inconsistencies

Most cases of invalid responding can be resolved by urging, reinstructing, explaining, and retesting (McCanna & DeLapa, 1981; Schlauch, Arnce, Olson, Sanchez & Doyle, 1996). The emphasis can be increased by asking the patient several times if he or she heard the signal heard, and suggesting that he or she will hear it soon (Nilo & Saunders, 1976).

Avoid confronting the patient (Bowdler & Rogers, 1989; Rintelmann & Schwan, 1999). It is wisest never to accuse the patient of or imply fakery. Provide a way to save face, an escape with honor (Maisami & Freeman, 1987; Pracy et al., 1996). Inform the patient that results are inconsistent or "don't make sense." Explain that this could be due to various factors, for instance misunderstanding directions, not felling well, or being nervous. Perhaps, they had misjudged the loudness and now they should respond to even very soft sounds. In any event, retesting is necessary. You can point out that more elaborate tests would resolve the inconsistencies but they are time-consuming and costly. Another try using the regular tests might make the special tests unnecessary. Realistically, time may not allow for retesting during the same session or day (Coles, 2001).

In cases of compensation for damage from loud noise, one might say that their pattern is not like that normally seen from excessive sound exposure (Coles, 2001; Snyder, 2001). One could point out in a nonthreatening way that continued inconsistencies might need to be mentioned in a report, which may likely disqualify the person for benefits. In that way, patients have the opportunity to reconsider their responses and can be retested then. Although best not to confront, Martin (2009) mentioned that, in military cases, one could inform that falsifying results is a violation of a military code of behavior and grounds for court martial. However, he warns of the risk of psychological trauma to a veteran, so this tactic must be used very prudently.

Auditory Processing Disorders

As indicated earlier, auditory processing disorders (APD) are mentioned as a possible factor in inconsistent responding. Hasbrouck's (1989) study led him to recommend that patients with FEHL be evaluated for an auditory perceptual disorder. This writer sees two problems with that recommendation. First, because there is little evidence that a significant proportion of persons who present FEHL have auditory perceptual disorders, testing all patients for APD would result in enormous overreferrals at a cost of worry, time, and money for low yield. Second, as others have asserted, when a patient exhibits FEHL, attention should be diverted away from hearing so as not to further reinforce the patient's notion of having a hearing problem. Yet, evaluating for an APD focuses attention on hearing. Obviously, if there is sufficient question of a processing disorder, the person should be referred.

Modifications

As a general rule, standard methods and materials should be used during pure-tone and speech audiometry with all patients. However, when FEHL complicates matters, modifications can be more effective. One could cast the matter as being unconventional with conventional audiometry. In doing the unconventional, it may seem that, whatever the usual approach is, do the opposite. A few "opposites" have been mentioned already: starting with speech instead of tones, and beginning at a very low level and ascending instead of presenting a few presumed suprathreshold stimuli and descending. Other tactics that run counter to usual procedure are alternating between tones and speech, changing frequency often to tones a few octaves away, and switching between ears many times. A further deviation from the norm is to have both the bone-conduction and air-conduction headsets in place at the same time in order to shift quickly between air- and bone-conducted signals (correcting for the low-frequency occlusion effect). The goals are to upset any loudness reference, check for consistency, and search for patterns.

Such unsystematic techniques require adroitness, not only in handling the controls, but also in keeping track of responses and no-responses, whether for tones or speech. For each stimulus presentation, this audiologist "keeps score," plotting various symbols on the audiogram, such as (+) for a response, (−) for no response, S for Speech, and B for unmasked bone conduction (symbols for right ear on the left of the frequency axis and left ear results on the right side, as is done with usual bone-conduction symbol placement). The point of such nontraditional coding is to obtain a "scatter plot" of responses to see if a pattern emerges that could be the basis of threshold estimates. If confident enough in the estimates, the traditional Xs and Os can be drawn on the audiogram to show them.

The finished product may show just a few Os and Xs at different frequencies (and not necessarily the same frequencies for each ear) with one or two unmasked bone conduction "thresholds." Instead of being a sign of deficient or ineffective testing, such plots may actually reflect superior testing of a difficult patient and give a good picture of the patient's hearing. Understandably, some non-audiologists might be uncomfortable with such sparse results. People are used to seeing—and want to see—the familiar array of Os, Xs, and brackets at all frequencies, even though testing was best focused on a few specific thresholds. Sometimes no information is preferable to dubious information. Schools, third-party payers, and other agencies can deem the results unacceptable without thresholds displayed for right and left ears across frequencies, SRTs, and word recognition scores. Presumably, if such results could have been obtained, they would have been. The solution is a well-written report explaining the reasons for limited results. A good collegial relationship with an agency or physician creates understanding and trust when results are unavoidably incomplete.

Ascending-Descending Gap

As mentioned earlier, first suspicion of invalid results ought to prompt keeping signal levels quite low. However, in addition to using an ascending intensity to find thresholds, one can also use a descending signal from a level above where the patient had last responded. The reason is that false responders produce higher thresholds for descending than for ascending approaches, but valid responders yield the same thresholds (see Harris, 1958, in Chapter 2, Historical Aspects). Apparently, false responders cannot maintain the same loudness standard for signals that begin at high and at low levels, and are biased toward a higher stopping point when the start level is high. Threshold differences at 500 to 2000 Hz usually will be on the order of 25 dB, but even a gap greater than 5 dB is positive for FEHL (Harris, 1958). If one begins with an ascending threshold approach, then a second threshold is established by a descending approach, or vice versa, to see if there is a telltale gap typical of false responders (Cherry & Ventry, 1976).

Harris's approach can be shortened by using just 1000 Hz. An ascending run is made from 0 dB HL in 5-dB steps until a response, and then a descending run is made from a high level (e.g., 75 dB HL) until no response. With a criterion gap of least 10 dB, this test has good sensitivity and specificity, and testing can be accomplished in under 2 minutes with a basic audiometer (Woodford, Harris, Marquette, Perry, & Barnhart, 1997). This manual ascending-descending gap evaluation is highly effective with children, according to McCanna and DeLapa (1981). Using a gap criterion of 15 dB, all 21 of their children with FEHL had a positive result. The threshold discrepancy might be enhanced by using 2-dB steps (Snyder, 2001).

Schlauch et al. (1996) compared ascending and descending speech thresholds on a group of normal hearing subjects who were instructed to feign a hearing loss. SRTs obtained by ascending runs averaged 9 dB lower than SRTs obtained by descending runs; the ascending SRTs were also 10 dB lower than the ascending pure tone averages. Schlauch et al. (1996) also compared *ascending SRTs* to *descending tone thresholds* on normal-hearing feigners and on persons with genuine hearing impairment. The feigning group had an average gap of 42 dB, and no case had a difference less than 19 dB (SRT lower). In contrast, the impaired group had a PTA-SRT difference of only 1.6 dB. In short, combining the ascending SRT and descending pure-tone approaches maximizes the difference between speech and tone thresholds. Schlauch et al. (1996) recommended this combination as a fast, effective screening test for high-risk groups and also as a way at the end of the evaluation to verify accuracy, in case (unknown to the clinician) a patient had produced false thresholds. Because this procedure necessarily involves a high-level signal, one can keep testing brief by using only the pure-tone average of 500 and 1000 Hz and a criterion of 10 dB for the PTA-SRT difference. If positive, subsequent threshold searches should be by ascending approaches only. Using short-duration tones minimizes the sense of loudness. As mentioned above, small increments of 2 dB might magnify any gap.

Lengthened Off Time

Using a standard audiometer, Martin, Martin, and Champlin (2000) examined combining the ascending-descending comparisons with different signal timings as a screening tool for false hearing loss. The temporal patterns were: continuously on (CON), a pulsed tone with standard off time (SOT) of 250 ms, and a pulsed tone with a lengthened off time (LOT) of 700 ms. Normal hearing subjects first responded normally and then simulated a hearing loss. The mean ascending-descending gap for the normal responding condition was 0.6 dB and for the simulated loss condition was 15.3 dB. The simulated threshold levels from the descending SOT and LOT were generally worse than the ascending CON thresholds. With a gap criterion of more than 10 dB, the CON-SOT-LOT procedure was sensitive and specific and only took 2 to 3 minutes. However, the authors recommended avoiding predictable patterns by using different off times, random ascending-descending approaches, and different starting intensities and rates of change.

Silent Control Periods

Among the various ways to check validity is using silent epochs to see if the patient makes false-positive responses. True responders probably will make a few, but pseudoresponders rarely make them. Chaiklin and Ventry (1965) found silent control periods of 30 seconds to be effective. They felt that, if patients gave false positive responses, they were about as likely to do so in the first 30 seconds as in the second 30 seconds of a 1-minute period. In this author's opinion, probably no more than 20 seconds is both effective and practical. The risk is that, the longer the interstimulus intervals, the more likely are other difficulties (e.g., excessive false responses in true patients). Ultimately, how often and how long those periods should be is a matter of clinical judgment.

Occlusion Effect

For unilateral hearing loss, Thompson and Denman (1970) proposed a quick and easy screening test that takes advantage of the occlusion effect. They had 10 normal hearers feign a total, right-ear hearing loss. When there was just a bone oscillator on the good (left) side, the subjects responded, but when the oscillator was on the poor (right) side, they almost never responded. Next, when the bone oscillator was placed on the good side and an earphone placed on the poor ear, subjects almost never responded to low-frequency signals. The reason is that, by the occlusion effect, the low frequencies were shifted to the poor ear, and subjects were to deny hearing in that ear. That outcome is positive for FEHL, because, if the loss were genuine, putting an earphone on an impaired ear would have no effect. Finally, when the oscillator was on the poor side and an earphone on the good ear, all subjects responded to low frequencies (but not to high frequencies) because the occlusion effect made the low frequencies more prominent in the good ear. The results for low frequencies can be summarized this way:

Mastoid	Occlusion	Response	Reason
good side	none	yes	testing good side
poor side	none	no	testing poor side
good side	phone on poor ear	no	signal shifted to poor side
poor side	phone on good ear	yes	signal shifted to good side

No doubt, a low-frequency signal could also be delivered by a tuning fork or a handheld BC oscillator, and an ear canal could be occluded with a finger. This is similar to the Bing Test, in which a tuning fork is placed on the skull vertex, one ear is alternately closed and opened, and the patient is asked if the sound changes location or loudness (it should when occluded if ears are normal in accordance with the Weber effect).

Tactics with Children

Miller, Fox, and Chan (1968) suggested three modifications to pure tone testing with children: (1) indicating when a descending, continuously-on tone was no longer heard, (2) judging if one tone of a pair was louder than the other while the tone pairs were gradually lowered in intensity until no response, and (3) responding to tones with "yes" or "no." Only the last one has remained in use.

In the yes-no test, children are instructed to say "yes" when they hear the tone and "no" when they do not. Some children do not see the incongruity of reacting to a supposedly inaudible sound by saying "no." The success of the test depends on the child responding right after the signal presentation and also on not responding when there is no signal or if it is below the child's true threshold (Frank, 1976). Martin's (2009) approach is to begin at the audiometer's lowest limit and raise intensity in 5-dB steps; he finds the test surprisingly effective (as does this author). Some children spontaneously adopt a "no" response. Audiograms showing normal hearing have been plotted based on credible "no" responses.

Dixon and Newby (1959) successfully assessed children's hearing by having them count the number of tones, when the usual hand-raise response was not credible. Ross (1964) improved on this technique with the variable intensity pulse count method (VIPCM). The task is presented as one of counting ability. The child is instructed to count how many tones are heard in a series of one to six tones. Initially, a few series of tones are presented above admitted thresholds to be sure the child can perform the task. Then, the intensity of one of the tones is given at 10 to 15 dB below the admitted threshold, and the other tones are given above threshold in short succession. A correct answer means the child heard the weaker tone. The intensity and number of tones are varied at random, one or more tones given below the admitted threshold interspersed with one or more tones above admitted threshold. Intensity is varied until the lowest level of three consecutive correct responses is found. If well timed and consistent, even incorrect answers can be indicative of hearing (Dixon & Newby, 1959). When a child says nothing during silent periods but says a number after a tone series, even if wrong, it is very likely that some of the series was heard. A wrong answer might be because the tones happen to be near true threshold and are difficult to detect. Or a child might make deliberate errors as a way of fabricating false results. Either way, incorrect answers can be helpful by their timing and consistency.

Hosoi et al. (1999) used "suggestion audiometry" on 20 children aged 8 to 16 years who had been identified as having false hearing losses, 12 bilateral and 8 unilateral. Each child was told that hearing would improve by using a hearing aid during the testing. A behind-the-ear aid was put in place on the ear but not turned on and had no tubing or ear tip, and then audiometry was performed. Next, the hearing aid was removed and the subjects were tested again. All but four showed a significant change. The suggestion produced an average pure-tone improvement of 26 dB, and a number of children had changes beyond 60 dB. The SRT showed less change, about 10 dB, but the SRT resulted in a more accurate estimate of the true threshold probably because the initial SRT was much closer to threshold to begin with.

Tips and Tricks

Few articles or book chapters devote attention to the variations and subtleties of testing or to the role of the clinician as a situation manager, not just as a test performer. This section has a list of tips and tricks based on experience and literature. The main sources were Brockman and Hoversten (1960), Campanelli (1963), McCanna and DeLapa (1981), Nilo and Saunders (1976), and Snyder (2001). For ease of reading, we have dispensed with citations. Most of the tips can be adapted to both adults and children. The categories below are for organization and convenience and should not be thought of as separate units. The tips are different possibilities to weave into a session. Finally, some acting skill definitely increases the effectiveness of these tips and tricks, or even makes them possible.

At the Start

- If you are suspicious during history taking, suggest one or two strange or illogical symptoms, because a false patient may respond in the affirmative.
- Merely using physiologic test instrumentation at the outset, such as immittance recorders and OAE screeners, probably discourages deceptive behavior.
- Say to patients that the above measurements will "tell a lot about your hearing."

- Have the patient see the results appear: an acoustic reflex meter's needle deflections, an indicator of "yes" or "pass," or tracings displayed with reference to a normal pattern.

Signal Variations

- Use warble or pulsed tones without warning or explanation, as they might result in a different reaction and help upset loudness memory.
- Give more than one tone or word at the same dB interval.
- Use a low level of informal conversation, for example, 30 dB, before actual tests (or select level based on observed pretesting ability), because the initial level serves as a loudness reference.
- Resist the temptation to increase intensity beyond 40 dB until all other efforts fail (but keep in mind that not responding or patient confusion could be because the signals are truly subthreshold.)

Exploit Suggestibility

- Use a tone of voice and words that imply expectation; people tend to behave in the direction in which they are expected to behave.
- Use explicit expectation: "You'll hear this one, so you'll raise your hand when you do."
- Introduce pure tone audiometry in a casual manner, remarking, "These tones are easy to hear."
- When a change in frequency or a shift to warble tones, say "here's an easier one."
- If reasonably confident that the signal is audible but there is no response, try, "I know you can hear this one; sure, go ahead, that's right; raise your hand."

- Blame the equipment. Feign that there was a problem (e.g., ear phone not plugged in; plug it in and assure that now the patient will hear it just fine).

Clinician Technique

- Constantly coax, cajole, and compliment.
- Direct some pretended treatment to the ears (e.g., removing some wax or even tympanometry) with suggestion that will hear better; this also gives an "escape."
- Look surprised, confused, or frustrated, if no response.
- Encourage response to pure tones by raising your own hand.
- Give a surprise command or rebuke (judiciously) below supposed threshold, and watch response: "Raise your hand higher;" or "No, please don't do that!"
- Use low-level, offhand remarks or questions, such as "You can take the earphones off now." "Did you say that you used to shoot guns?" "What grade are you in?"
- Positive reinforcement: verbal ("good job," "that's right") and nonverbal (nod approval, smile, and so forth) to affirm a response.
- Prompt by pointing to ear as if telling to listen; gesture that the next sound will be very soft.
- Using a soft or normal voice, begin a sentence or question that calls for a response while facing the patient and then turn away for some task while finishing the utterance with some information-bearing words, for example, "I know your shop was loud. Did you (turning to get the headset, move a chair, reach for some item) have to wear (faced away) eye protection also?" Demonstrating better hearing is especially helpful when another person is observing.

- Start a conversation in the patient room and continue it when in the control booth at a low level in the sound field to give the impression of chatting rather than testing.
- Feign a pretext at a soft level of needing some extra information while acting as if getting ready to start (e.g., "How do you spell your first name?")
- Insert what seems an extraneous, incidental remark and watch reaction, such as, "By the way, I like your jacket," or "OK, just relax for a moment while I write down some results."
- Use intonation that expresses reassurance, expectation, confidence that, "yes, you can."
- Engage the person in low-level conversation about a topic that the person is interested; the person may be caught off guard. "So, you're a hunter. I used to go for quail. What do you hunt?"

Response

- Consider introducing button pressing as an alternative response under the ploy of being "easier." To some patients, this seems logical and makes the response more concrete. It also gives the false responder an "out."
- Accept minimal responses if consistent, like starting to raise a hand but stops.
- If the patient responds to a spondee after a delay or with an intonation of guessing, capitalize on it with acceptance and reassurance, and advise that can be more confident.
- When a wide range of responses makes it difficult to find a 50% correct level, consider accepting a lower rate, provided responses seemed valid.
- Try an ear-pointing response; present as a game or task of identifying which ear, not as a hearing test.

- Use ear pointing for a supposed equipment check. "I had some trouble with that left earphone; would you tell me if this sound is coming out of the left phone?" (The signal can be presented below admitted threshold to either ear.)

Speech Audiometry

- Seek a word recognition score at 30 dB in the sound field.
- If not responding, ask at the testing level, "Why didn't you say the words?" or "Can't you hear the words?" This creates expectation. Also, a reply indicates better hearing.
- During speech audiometry, waiting a few seconds can elicit a response.
- If client gives half word responses, tell them that if they hear half the word to say the whole word as was done during the practice.
- During ascending SRT, intersperse comments such as, "I know the words seem soft, but go ahead and give it a try." "It's OK to guess, if you think you got it."

What Not To Do and What To Do

Don't: convey judgment or irritation.

Instead: convey empathy; the sense of a friend, not enemy.

Don't: corner or trap.

Instead: seek ways of eliciting cooperation, rather than alienating.

Don't: respond in kind, if the patient becomes angry or hostile.

Instead: maintain a calm attitude and remain objective.

Don't: get pulled into an adversarial situation/argument, if a patient says, "Are you calling me a liar?"

Instead: reply to the effect, "Sorry, you must have misunderstood. Maybe I explained it badly. I'm just saying that the results seem out of the ordinary and I don't know why. The sooner we get this straightened out, the sooner things can proceed for your benefits."

Summary

Conventional behavioral procedures have the advantages of simplicity, convenience, and low cost, as well as being truly direct tests of hearing. If test discrepancies arise, they usually can be resolved by reinstructing, encouraging, and retesting. Otherwise, a good rule is to proceed with speech audiometry. Whether testing by speech or tones, use low signal levels, ascending intensity, and small dB steps. Watch for subtle body and facial gestures, which may be indications of having heard the signal. When testing does not go easily or results seem invalid, it is best to be organized and do the "basics." At the same time, it is important to recognize when and how to depart "from standard procedures, which experienced clinicians probably do" (Martin, Champlin, & McCreery, 2001, p. 63). Key characteristics are being flexible, unconventional, and creative.

Notice the absence of a recommended test sequence or protocol. This audiologist is not in favor of them because with FEHL the situation is so spontaneous and fluid. The idea of following a predetermined plan of action runs counter to the idea of making moment-to-moment choices. Instead, this chapter offers a set of principles as a framework for making effective decisions. Chapter 7, which follows, stays in the realm of behavioral approaches by considering procedures developed specifically for FEHL.

Chapter 7

SPECIAL BEHAVIORAL TESTS

Identification of a functional hearing problem may be the simplest job for the audiologist to learn, while resolution of hearing levels may be the most difficult.

—Hopkinson, 1973, p. 188

Introduction

The last chapter dealt with conventional behavioral tests and their modifications. This chapter continues with behavioral tests designed specifically for use in FEHL, namely, the Stenger tests, the Story test, and the Falconer lipreading test.

Stenger Test

Bases

The Stenger test is based on the Stenger principle, which is "when two tones of the same frequency are introduced simultaneously into both ears, only the louder tone will be perceived" (Mendel, Danhauer, & Singh, 1999; Stach, 2003). Actually, the effect applies to any sounds that are identical at the two ears. Sometimes, instead of loudness, the Stenger principle is stated in terms of the ear receiving the greater intensity. These are not always the same thing. Generally, greater intensity will result in greater loudness, but hearing loss can alter that relationship. Some examples will help illustrate this effect

Normal hearing: If a normal-hearing person is presented with a 10-dB HL tone to one ear and a 40-dB tone to the other ear, the person will be aware only of the tone in the ear where the signal is stronger and therefore louder.

Bilateral hearing impairment: If a person has a 30-dB hearing impairment in both ears, and a 40-dB HL tone is delivered to one ear and a 70-dB tone to the other ear, the person will perceive only the tone in the ear where the signal is stronger. In both this and the previous case, the sensation levels are 10 dB in one ear and 40 dB in the other ear.

Unilateral conductive hearing impairment: If a person has a unilateral 30-dB conductive hearing impairment and if identical tones of 40 dB HL are presented to each ear, the person will hear the tone only in the normal ear. The reason is because the SL in the normal ear is 40 dB while the SL in the poor ear is only 10 dB and therefore much softer. This is an example of the Stenger effect in which *the same intensities result in different loudnesses.* The effect of the conductive loss can be offset by equalizing the sensation levels, for example in this case, delivering a 40-dB HL tone to the normal ear and a 70-dB HL tone to the poor ear. The person will not hear a tone in just one ear to the exclusion of the other, because the Sensation Levels are 30 dB in each ear. This is an example of *different intensities resulting in the same loudness.*

Unilateral cochlear hearing impairment: If a person has a 30-dB cochlear impairment in one ear, and tones of 40 dB HL are presented to both ears, the person will hear the tone only in the normal ear. The reason is the large difference in SLs: 40 dB in the normal ear but only 10 dB in the poor ear. So far, this is exactly the same as the above unilateral conductive loss. However, if much stronger tones are presented to each ear, say 80 dB HL, loudness would be about the same in the two ears due to recruitment, and a tone would not be lateralized to either ear. Thus, even when there is a hearing impairment, loudness equivalence can depend on absolute intensity. The 40-dB signal level is an example of *different loudnesses at low intensity*, and the 80-dB level is an example of *equal loudness at high intensity* for the same hearing loss.

Instrumentation and Ear Difference

Whether tones or speech, the signals must be identical in every way in order to be indistinguishable at the two ears. For tones, the signal should come from one oscillator (or two synchronized oscillators) for identical frequency and phase and be presented by one switch for simultaneous on and off. Any such concerns are avoided in the speech version of the Stenger, because the signal has a single source, whether live or recorded. Regardless of the type of signal, there must be two hearing level attenuators for independent control of the intensities going to the two earphones. Virtually all modern diagnostic audiometers have the capabilities of meeting these requirements.

In a normal-hearing person, if the signal strength reaching the two ears is the same, the perception is in the middle of the head. Even a difference of 1 dB makes the sound seem to shift slightly toward the ear where the signal is stronger and therefore louder. As the difference increases, so also does the sense of laterality. When the ear difference reaches 10 dB, the perception is purely in one ear (Hamill & Price, 2008). One can experience the sensation of shifting sound location by listening through earphones and varying the right-left loudness balance.

Tone Stenger Test Procedures

The Stenger test (1907), originally performed with tuning forks, must be the oldest test designed to identify FEHL that is still in use. It is applicable to either unilateral or asymmetric losses that have at least a 40-dB difference in thresholds between the ears. The procedure is to present a tone 10 dB above threshold to the "good" ear and simultaneously an identical tone 10 dB below apparent threshold to the "poor" ear. If the poor-ear threshold is genuine, the patient will respond, because, although the tone in the poor ear is inaudible, the tone in the good ear is still audible. This is known as a negative Stenger and confirms the hearing loss. In contrast, if hearing in the poor ear is actually normal but the patient wishes to disguise the fact, the patient will hear the tone just in the poor ear and not respond. The signal in the good ear is not perceived because the signal in the poor ear is stronger and therefore louder; the patient denies hearing it by not responding. This is a positive Stenger, which means that hearing in the poor ear must be significantly better than the alleged threshold. Note that it is the *absence of response* that is the positive result.

Now and then, an invalid responder may continue to respond even when they no longer perceive the signal in the better ear. An example would be a calculating or test-wise person supposing that a tone is simultaneously going to the good ear. Hence, when the Stenger is negative, a way to check the outcome is to withhold occasionally the signal to the good ear. A response would mean that the person hears the signal in the bad ear, even though it is supposedly below threshold, which is a variant positive result. Should that be the case, the clinician should continue seeking a threshold in that ear. If the patient reverts to the tactic of not responding, one can double-check validity by presenting the tone just to the good ear. Failure to respond shows invalid performance, because the signal in the good ear is still 10 dB above threshold.

With a few quick changes in the audiometer's settings, the Stenger test can easily be interjected into ongoing pure-tone audiometry without the patient being aware of anything different about the testing. An asymmetric situation can be screened for validity in less than half a minute (Hattler & Schuchman, 1971). Thus, there is no reason not to apply the Stenger any time there is a question of unilateral/asymmetrical FEHL.

A highly valuable attribute of the Stenger test is its ability to quantify true hearing. To do so, the tone to the good ear is kept at 10 dB SL. Because the Stenger test was already positive when the poor-ear tone was 10 dB below admitted threshold, one could continue with a tone 20 dB below that threshold. If no response, reduce the signal in 10-dB steps until the patient responds. Or one could follow an ascending approach as Martin (2009) suggests, starting at 0 dB HL with 5-dB increments until the patient does not respond. Regardless of the starting point, the intensity to the poor ear is adjusted until the lowest level of "no response" is established. The lack of a response means that the tone in the bad ear is loud enough to interfere with hearing the tone in the good ear. The lowest hearing level of "no response" is the minimum contralateral interference level (MCIL). The final step in predicting genuine threshold is subtracting 10 dB from the MCIL to correct for the level above threshold in the good ear. By subtracting the SL in the good ear from that level in the poor ear, one can estimate true threshold within 5 to 15 dB. A sensation level at the good ear of 10 dB typically has been utilized, so that the signal is definitely audible but low enough to make the test most effective. A finer resolution of threshold can be sought by conducting the test at only 5 or even 0 dB SL in the good ear and then subtracting that SL from the MCIL. These low levels are usable, as most people respond consistently during conventional audiometry at 5 or 0 dB SL. If such low signal levels are used, the Stenger could be tried on persons having only a 20-dB ear difference between admitted thresholds (Robinette & Gaeth, 1972).

If using the ascending approach, there may be merit in starting at 10 dB HL (instead of 0 dB HL) and going up in 10-dB steps (instead of 5 dB), so the patient does not become confused or suspicious because of the repeated, unchanging tone in the good ear. For example, if the person's true threshold were 25 dB, going up from 0 dB in 5-dB increments might take seven steps before the first "no response" as opposed to maybe three steps, if starting at 10 dB HL with 10-dB increments. In any event, there is little difference in efficiency between the ascending and descending approaches (Peck & Ross, 1970). Perhaps more important than an ascending or descending approach is performing the test skillfully to take full advantage of the Stenger effect. As Martin (2009) points out, if the clinician is not experienced in administration, repetitive patterns of tone presentations "may betray the intentions of the test" to a perceptive patient.

Speech Stenger Test Procedures

The speech Stenger test operates on the same principles and in the same way as the pure-tone version with the obvious difference of using speech in stead of pure tones. First, SRTs are established in the usual fashion. To verify the SRT in the poor ear, spondaic words are presented at 10 dB SL in the good ear and at 10 dB below tentative SRT in the poor ear. If the patient repeats a few words, it is a negative speech Stenger and corroborates the SRT. However, a cunning patient might repeat words, having figured out that words could be going to the good ear. As a check, the signal to the good ear can be withheld from time to time, and the true patient would not say any words. Otherwise, if the patient fails to repeat a few words, one can search for the MCIL as is done with tones. Words in the good ear are kept at 5 or 10 dB SL, and signal intensity to the poor ear is changed in descending or ascending fashion until the lowest level is established of failing to repeat two or more spondees. That level is the MCIL for speech. Speech MCILs can be found as low as 15 dB above the true SRT of the poor ear. An MCIL as low as 30 dB HL can be presumed to indicate normal hearing for speech (Martin, 2009). Threshold estimation is then accomplished by subtracting the sensation level in the good ear from the MCIL.

Employing monitored live voice allows greater flexibility and creativity. One can use informal speech in addition to or in place of spondees, so it does not seem like testing. The clinician can give some off-hand instruction, ask questions, or make comments all while varying the SLs in each ear. As with conventional audiometry, the Stenger estimated speech threshold should be compared to the Stenger estimated tone threshold and the two should agree within 5 dB.

Hypothetical Case Examples

Table 7–1 gives several hypothetical examples of the Stenger test. They could apply to the tone or speech version. For simplicity, the right ear is always the "worse" ear, or if nearly symmetrical, the ear with the larger false component. "Good" and "bad" ear or similar terms refer to their supposed loss, not to their true hearing. Thus, the worse ear according to test results might actually hear as well or better than the good ear. Also, let us suppose that the test would not be positive unless the difference in sensation levels exceeds 10 dB. In other words, if the SLs at the two ears are within 10 dB, we will not suppose that the difference causes an inescapable perception of the signal on just one side or the other. The intention is to present various combinations of genuine and false hearing loss in the two ears to show the workings of the Stenger test. It is not practical to present every conceivable permutation of hearing loss.

To read Table 7–1, we must understand the 10 columns providing the information on the 10 (hypothetical) cases. Starting at the left, the first column, *Condition*, describes the person's audiologic situation. The next column, *True Threshold*, provides the person's genuine thresholds for right and left ears, although one would not know them at the time. Third is *Alleged Threshold*, the voluntary

Table 7–1. Explanation of the Stenger Test Through Hypothetical Sets of Alleged Audiometric Thresholds

	True Threshold		Alleged Threshold		Overlay		Signal in dB HL		True SL					
Condition	R	L	R	L	R	L	R	L	R	L	SL Differ	Where Heard	Respond	Result +/–
Case 1. Valid unilateral HL	40	0	40	0	0	0	30	10	–10	10	–20	L	Yes	–
Case 2. Invalid unilateral HL	0	0	40	0	40	0	30	10	30	10	20	R	No	+
Case 3. Valid 30-dB asymmetry	70	40	70	40	0	0	60	50	–10	10	–20	L	Yes	–
Case 4. Invalid 40-dB asymmetry	40	40	80	40	40	0	70	50	30	10	20	R	No	+
Case 5. Invalid 30-dB asymmetry	40	40	70	40	30	0	60	50	20	10	10	M	?	X
Case 6. Invalid 40-dB asymmetry, small overlay	65	40	80	40	15	0	70	50	5	10	–5	M	?	X
Case 7. Invalid 20-dB asymmetry	25	40	60	40	35	0	50	50	25	10	15	R	No	+
Case 8. Symmetric unilateral overlay	0	50	50	50	50	0	40	60	40	10	30	R	No	+
Case 9. Invalid bilateral, asymmetric	0	0	50	20	50	20	40	30	40	30	10	X	?	X
Case 10. Bilateral HL mild bilateral overlay	50	30	75	50	25	20	65	60	15	30	–15	L	Yes	–

thresholds presented by the patient. The next column, *Overlay*, tells how much of the loss is false, if any; it is the difference between True Threshold and Alleged Threshold. The *Signal in dB HL* is the dial setting according to the Stenger test to present the signal 10 dB below the bad ear's alleged threshold and 10 dB above the good ear's alleged threshold. The *True SL* column shows the actual sensation level that results from the Stenger test, that is, the difference between the Signal in dB HL and the True Threshold. The *SL Differ* is the difference in sensation levels between the two ears; positive means the SL is higher in the bad ear than in the good ear and negative means the SL is lower in the bad ear. *Where Heard* is the ear in which the signal is likely to be perceived based on the difference in SL between the two ears (right, left, midline). The *Respond* column shows if the patient responds (yes, no, or unknown), given in which ear the sound was heard and the patient's willingness to acknowledge hearing in that ear. Finally, the *Result +/–* is the interpretation of the outcome as a positive Stenger (+), a negative Stenger (–) or uncertain (X).

Let's go through the first two cases step by step to follow how the Stenger test operates. These cases illustrate the workings of the test by using examples of a valid and an invalid unilateral hearing loss. Case 1 has a valid 40-dB hearing loss in the right ear. The alleged threshold equals the true threshold, so there is no overlay. Suppose that a clinician wants to verify the validity with the Stenger test. The clinician must present signals that are 10 dB below the poorer ear's alleged threshold and 10 dB above the better ear's threshold. In this case, the signal levels would be 30 dB in the right ear and 10 dB in the left ear. Because this is an example of a valid hearing loss, the true SLs are 10 dB below the threshold of the right ear and 10 dB above the threshold of the left ear. The SL difference of –20 dB means that the signal is definitely louder in the left ear; indeed, the signal is inaudible in the right ear so it could not interfere with hearing the signal in the left ear. The patient hears the signal in the left ear and responds. The patient's response is interpreted as a negative Stenger and says that the loss in the right ear must be valid.

Case 2 also presents a 40-dB hearing loss in the right ear but hearing is actually normal. The false portion (overlay) is 40 dB. The clinician applies the Stenger test by presenting signals that are 10 dB below the right ear's alleged threshold and 10 dB above the left ear's threshold. Thus, the signal level would be 30 dB HL in the right ear and 10 dB HL in the left ear, just as in Case 1. However, because hearing is actually normal, the true sensation levels are 30 dB in the right ear and 10 dB in the left ear. Because the SL is 20 dB higher in the right ear, the person hears the signal only in that ear. Wishing to present a hearing loss in the right ear, the person does not respond, which is classified as positive for invalid hearing loss. With this detailed background, the reader can read the simpler synopses of the remaining eight cases.

Case 3 is a genuine, asymmetric hearing loss with an ear difference of 30 dB. In administering the Stenger test, the only suprathreshold signal is in the better ear, so the patient responds, which is a negative Stenger.

Case 4 presents an asymmetric hearing loss but, in contrast to Case 3, the ear difference is due to an exaggeration by 40-dB in the worse ear. In applying the Stenger test, the actual SL to the worse ear is higher than the SL to the better ear, 30 dB versus 10 dB. The patient hears the signal in the worse ear but is unwilling to react to signals in the bad ear, so does not respond. The lack of response is a positive Stenger.

Case 5 is another invalid asymmetric hearing loss, although the false asymmetry is smaller because the overlay is smaller, 30 dB versus 40 dB in Case 4. The Stenger test signals result in similar sensation levels in the two ears. A patient probably would not hear the signal as being exclusively in one ear or the other. Hence, a person may or may not respond.

Case 6 is also meant to be contrasted to Case 4. Note that the alleged hearing thresholds are the same with a large, 40-dB asymmetry. However, the overlay in Case 4 is 40 dB whereas in this case it is only 15 dB (the worse ear really does have more hearing loss). As a result, the true sensation levels are within 5 dB. The patient likely would not have a definite perception of laterality. The point is that two patients with the same set of thresholds may have different Stenger outcomes because of different magnitudes of genuine or false loss.

Case 7 presents only a small ear difference of 20 dB. Unknown to the clinician, the patient actually has better hearing in the right ear than in the left ear, even though the right ear displays greater loss than the left ear. Once the test signals are calculated and applied, there is a significantly higher SL at the right ear. The patient would be aware of the signal in that ear and deny hearing it. The result is a positive Stenger despite a small ear difference.

Case 8 appears to have a symmetrical hearing loss of 50 dB. As such, it would not call for the Stenger test. However, this hypothetical patient has normal hearing in one ear and a true loss in the other ear. This is not such an implausible scenario. Imagine a person with one known bad ear, who wants to show that even the one good ear is not really a good ear in order to get compensation. If the Stenger test were given for this loss, the test signals would result in a high sensation level in the false ear and a low sensation level in the true ear, and the test would be positive. If there is a suspected large difference between ears despite identical thresholds, one could employ the Stenger.

Case 9 portrays a situation with normal hearing in both ears along with a large (50 dB) false loss in the bad ear and a small (20 dB) false loss in the better ear. The latter is enough to result in a higher signal level and SL. As a result the two SLs are not so dissimilar. Thus, just a small false portion in the better ear can make the test ineffective, even though there is a substantial ear difference (30 dB) and a large false loss (50 dB) in the bad ear.

In Case 10, there is a true bilateral hearing loss, which is moderate in the worse ear and mild in the better ear. There is also a small false component in each ear. Notice that the signal levels produce a 15-dB SL advantage in the better ear. Therefore, the patient would respond, and the test would be negative despite the 25-dB overlay in the worse ear. The true portion of the loss in the bad ear does not result in the signal level having a higher sensation level than if the loss were entirely false. On the other hand, the small overlay in the better ear requires an increase in the signal level to keep the signal 10 dB above the voluntary threshold, which results in a sensation level higher than the supposed 10 dB in the better ear.

Critique of the Stenger

The effectiveness of the Stenger tests is influenced be various factors, chief among them the professed interaural threshold difference. Using an ear difference criterion of 20 dB or more, Ventry and Chaiklin (1965a) found the Stenger tests were less efficient detectors of FEHL than either the pure tone test-retest relationship or the spondee threshold-PTA relationship. The Stenger tests identified only about 42% of their subjects. Applying a criterion of ear asymmetry of 15 dB, Hattler and Schuchman (1971) found that the tone Stenger test was applicable in 57% of all their cases and detected only 48% of the FEHL cases, quite close to the 42% found by Ventry and Chaiklin.

Kinstler, Phelan, and Lavender (1970, 1972) replicated the Ventry-Chaiklin study. Even though they used the same ear difference criterion of 20 dB or more, the tone and speech Stenger tests each identified close to 82% of cases. They attributed the greater effectiveness to the larger true interaural differences in most of their cases.

According to Ventry and Chaiklin (1965a), the two variables that most affect the efficiency of the Stenger tests are: (a) the size of the alleged interaural sensitivity difference and (b) the size of the invalid component in the worse ear. Results are highly likely to be positive when both are greater than 40 dB. Also, results are highly likely to be negative if the better ear had even a mild (<25 dB) false component.

The ascending and descending approaches to administering the Stenger test were compared in detection rate and threshold predictability (Peck & Ross, 1970). Thirty-five, normal-hearing adults were instructed to make the tester believe that they could hear nothing in one ear. Each mode of administration identified all subjects as presenting false hearing loss, and the minimum interference levels differed by only 1.3 dB (testing was in 2-dB steps). The combined average minimum contralateral interference level was 8.4 dB above genuine thresholds, which was strikingly close to the 10 dB-SL tone in the better ear. Ninety-five percent of the subjects had MCILs within 14 dB of their true thresholds in the better ear.

Durmaz, Karahatay, Satar, Birkent, and Hidir (2009) evaluated the efficacy of the pure-tone Stenger test by calculating its sensitivity, specificity, and predictive values. The subjects were 200 military recruits presenting questionable profound or total hearing loss in one ear. The validating criterion was click ABR threshold measurements. Per the ABR, 190 persons were confirmed as truly having profound hearing losses. The Stenger test agreed in 189 cases, giving a specificity of 99.4%. Specificity is the probability of correctly identifying persons who do not have the condition. In this study the condition is FEHL, so specificity refers to the ability of the test to identify those who do not have FEHL. The remaining 10 candidates were classified as having FEHL, in that their behavioral results showing profound loss were worse than their ABR thresholds of 95 dB to 30 dB nHL. Of those 10, the Stenger identified 7, equaling a sensitivity of 70%. Sensitivity is the probability of correctly identifying persons who do have the condition.

The Stenger's positive predictive value was 87.5% (7 confirmed by ABR out of 8 positive cases by the Stenger). Positive predictive value is the probability that patients with a positive test result are correctly categorized. The test's negative predictive value was 98.4% (192 negative by the Stenger; of those, 189 ears were also negative by ABR, thus true negatives, and 3 were positive by ABR, thus false negatives). Negative predictive value is the probability that patients with a negative test result are correctly categorized.

Diplacusis has been mentioned as possibly precluding applying the Stenger test. Diplacusis is an abnormal condition of hearing two different tones for a single frequency. There are two types: diplacusis monauralis and diplacusis binauralis. Diplacusis monauralis is hearing two different tones or sounds in one ear from a single stimulus. Diplacusis binauralis is hearing different pitches in the two ears from the same stimulus. Because the Stenger tests depend on the signals sounding the same, either type of diplacusis could enable the patient to separate sounds in the two ears and nullify the Stenger effect. These problems are thought to be overcome by using speech in place of tones, although conceivably the distortion cause by an auditory disorder might make speech sound different in the two ears.

In the only study of the effect of diplacusis on the Stenger test, Robinette and Gaeth (1972) trained four normal hearers and four persons with unilateral sensorineural hearing losses and diplacusis in ways to defeat the tone Stenger test. The normal hearers had tuning mismatches between the ears of no more than 20 Hz, whereas the impaired subjects had mismatches of 83 to 146 Hz. Initially, the normal hearing and the hearing-impaired subjects did not differ in their ability to "beat" the test. With practice, the normal group improved in invalidating the test but the unilateral loss group did not. The authors concluded that diplacusis does not automatically rule out trying the tone Stenger test. Also, the first presentations are probably the most valid ones before patients learn how to recognize binaural presentations. Robinette and Gaeth felt that the test should not be considered "unbeatable" because, at least with some experience, normal listeners can improve in defeating the test.

A reasonable question is, To what extent does sophistication about tests reduce their effectiveness? As early as 1949, Taylor (1949) assessed that issue by teaching a group of normal-hearing subjects about the workings of the Stenger tests and ways to invalidate them. Practice greatly reduced test effectiveness; however, varying how the tests were administered helped maintain their accuracy.

Similarly, Monro and Martin (1977) assessed the effects of sophistication on measures to detect FEHL: pure-tone Stenger test, tone DAF, PTA-SRT discrepancy, and ascending-descending gap. They asked young, normal-hearing adults to feign a unilateral, moderate to severe hearing loss. One group was merely given standard instructions for a hearing test. Another group had the underlying principles of each test explained to them, and were told how they could "beat" the test. The third group had the foregoing information plus practice before taking the actual tests. DAF was moderately affected, and the SRT-PTA and ascending-descending gaps were substantially affected by sophistication. The tone Stenger screening test was not influenced and remained 100% effective in detecting false hearing loss.

Using much the same research method, Martin and Shipp (1982) studied the effects of sophistication on tests used to establish true thresholds: the tone and speech Stenger test and the tone DAF test. Given just standard instructions, the average positive result by DAF occurred about 4 dB above true threshold and the average positive result by the Stenger tests occurred 12 dB above true threshold. Not only was the DAF test a close indicator of true threshold, but the level of sophistication did not affect DAF threshold predictions. On the other hand, sophistication and practice helped subjects portray greater hearing loss on the two Stenger tests, on average by about 17 dB. On the tone Stenger, instructing was a slight help but practice was a bigger help. The reverse was true of the speech Stenger in that instruction was a greater help than the training. Because clinicians usually do not know a patient's level of sophistication with the Stenger tests, they must remember that those tests are not foolproof identifiers of threshold.

These and other studies had used normal-hearing subjects who were instructed to feign hearing loss. Ventry (1976a) cautioned against generalizing from normal-hearing simulators to real patients with FEHL, because their similarities may be outweighed by their differences: motivation, experience with hearing tests, listening strategies, and coexisting organic hearing disorder. He urged using subjects with confirmed false loss. Martin and Monro (1976) agreed that caution was in order but defended employing research subjects, because with actual patients, one cannot manipulate the controlled variables, such as listener sophistication. It is uncertain—and perhaps unknowable—to what extent actual false responders and test subjects told to feign a hearing loss yield different results. Perhaps, each has its unique value in this sort of research.

Studies finding different degrees of Stenger effectiveness may not be in conflict but instead may reflect the applicability of the tests to the size of the difference between the supposed thresholds. In fact, viewed from the standpoint of differences in thresholds between the ears, the studies are very much in agreement. When the ear differences presented were 40 dB or more, the Stenger tests were highly accurate detectors of FEHL and also quite good threshold estimators within 10 to 15 dB. When the differences between the supposed thresholds were 20 dB or less, the tests were not dependable.

Factors in Outcome

The Stenger test is most effective when there is an ear difference in voluntary thresholds of 40 dB or more. If the 40-dB ear difference is false, the result will be positive (see Cases 2 and 4 in Table 7–1). If the 40-dB ear difference is partly or completely genuine, the result will be negative or ambiguous (see Case 6 in Table 7–1).

In effect, a false component at the bad ear increases the true sensation level at the bad ear. In stead of a supposed 10-dB SL signal, as the test calls for, because the false threshold is higher than the true threshold, the actual SL is higher than −10 dB. If the overlay is 20 dB, then the resultant SL is 10 dB, not −10 dB, as it would be if the entire loss were genuine. The larger the false portion in the bad ear, the greater the sensation level. The greater the sensation level in the bad ear, the more likely is a positive result. As for the good ear, even a mild false portion adds to the sensation level in that ear. A higher SL in the good ear reduces the difference in SLs between ears, thereby increasing the chance of a negative result.

An organic hearing loss in either ear has little effect on detecting a unilateral false component (see Cases 4 and 7 in Table 7–1), although a genuine hearing loss in the good ear makes the Stenger test appear less applicable (as in Case 8 in Table 7–1). Because true hearing loss does not raise the signal's SL beyond 10 dB, it does not affect the true interaural SL difference. As long as there is a 40-dB false component in the bad ear, the Stenger test will still be positive (Cases 2, 4, 7, and 8 in Table 7–1). Nonetheless an organic loss in either ear could be accompanied by recruitment, tinnitus, and/or diplacusis, which would increase the chances of an incorrect negative.

The reason that the admitted threshold difference must be 40 dB is because the test calls for −10 dB SL to the bad ear and +10 dB SL to the good ear. Reducing the signal level by 10 dB to the bad ear and raising the signal by 10 dB to the good ear (relative to supposed thresholds) makes for a 20-dB smaller difference in sound levels between the two ears. As a result, a threshold difference of 40 dB is transformed into a test signal difference of 20 dB. However, if hearing were actually normal in each ear, the 20-dB signal difference would also be a 20-dB SL difference, which would be sufficient to cause complete lateralization. A signal level difference less than 20 dB would not unquestionably cause the sound to be shifted entirely to one ear. In effect, the test itself cancels out 20 dB of any initial threshold difference. We might call this the Stenger 20-dB cancellation effect. Furthermore, because thresholds are measured in 5-dB intervals and normal threshold variability is within 5 dB, a tone of "10 dB SL" might be something less than 10 dB SL. Therefore, the initial difference must be large enough to override these factors and assure the full Stenger effect.

Summary of the Stenger Test

To summarize, the Stenger test, with few exceptions, will be positive when there is a false difference between ears of at least 40 dB regardless of any other factors. False portions influence the outcome, but organic portions generally do not. Apart from diplacusis or familiarity with the test, the outcome ultimately is determined by the interaural difference in sensation levels, which relates to any false portions in the two ears. If the difference in SL is greater than 10 to 15 dB favoring the bad ear, the outcome very likely will be positive and indicate invalidity in the ear receiving the higher SL. Of course, all these parameters are unknown at the time of testing. The only thing known is the obtained thresholds. These various interactions may explain why some clinicians become disenchanted with the Stenger test or say that they don't have "much luck with it." If the test does not turn out positive (and the way the clinician had hoped or expected), it is for very good reason. The negative result informs the clinician that at least some of the hearing loss in the bad ear is genuine.

The minimum criterion of a 40-dB interaural difference is sometimes described as a limitation, but it is not so much a limitation as a statement of applicability. That the Stenger test is not applicable when threshold differences are less than 40 dB is no more a limitation than saying that EOAE testing is not applicable when there is a conductive hearing loss and a flat tympanogram. Despite any shortcomings, the evidence says that, when applicable, the Stenger tests are rapid and accurate, hardly matched among behavioral tests for detecting false thresholds and estimating true thresholds.

Under favorable conditions—naïve patient, normal hearing, large alleged interaural difference, experienced clinician, and proper equipment—the Stenger test is unbeatable. If some of those conditions are lacking, the Stenger test is less helpful or even useless. However, even if the difference in voluntary thresholds is less than 40 dB (as in Case 8 in Table 7-1), one can try the Stenger. If the results are positive, one has trustworthy information. If the results are negative, the possibility of some false hearing loss is not completely eliminated. Should there be lingering doubt as to legitimacy of the thresholds presented, one must use other procedures to corroborate or reject genuine hearing loss.

Story Tests

Story tests came about as a way to confirm unilateral false hearing losses. To do so, some parts of a story were fed to the good ear, and some parts to the poor ear in alternating fashion, and still other parts went to both ears simultaneously. The signal to the poor ear was kept 10 dB below the supposed threshold and the signal to the better ear 10 dB above threshold (similar to the Stenger test). The purpose of frequent shifts between either ear and both ears was to make it difficult to recall what information had been directed just to the poor ear. The patient then retold the story as much as possible. If the person mentioned anything that had been fed solely to the poor ear, one had evidence of ability to hear speech in that ear no worse than that signal level. Because the speech shifts or "swings" back and forth between ears, this approach often was referred to as the swinging story test (less often the swinging voice test).

Story tests require a two-channel audiometer to present different portions of a story through the speech circuit to either ear and to both ears. Stories were written so that each part could stand alone as its own story. A story had to be administered without gaps to ensure a sense of continuity, lest the patient become aware that the story is being shifted from ear to ear. Making the rapid changes while presenting the story via MLV requires considerable dexterity and sophistication (Martin, 1997). A prerecorded version makes the task easier (Martin, 2009).

In a modified version, Part 2 is not a separate story but rather a set of phrases which, when intermixed with Part 1, creates a much different story. In other words, if just Part 1 is heard, the story has one sense; if Part 2 is also heard, the story has quite a different meaning (e.g., china as in crockery, and China, the country) (Martin, 1997).

The Varying Intensity Story Test (VIST) is a revised approach that could be applied to either unilateral or bilateral FEHL and could give some estimate of threshold (Martin, Champlin, & Marchbanks, 1998). As described above, Part 1 had one story topic, and adding Part 2 made for an entirely different topic. Part 2 could be is administered through a range of 30 to 50 dB below admitted threshold, hence the varying intensity. If a patient shows awareness of the story formed by the combined Parts 1 and 2, the person must be able to hear speech at least at the test level of Part 2. When Martin, Champlin, and Marchbanks' (1998) normal-hearing subjects feigned a moderate unilateral hearing loss, most of them exhibited thresholds on the VIST that were 30 dB better than their stimulated thresholds. Even though the entire enterprise sounds rather elaborate, the VIST has been described as quick and easy (Martin, 2009). However, the VIST has not been evaluated on clinical cases (Martin, 2009), and story tests have had a marginal role in evaluating FEHL. Also, astute patients might recognize the examiner's strategy and refuse to cooperate (Snyder, 2001).

Falconer's Lipreading Test

Falconer's (1966) "Lipreading" test is represented to the patient as a measure of lipreading ability, yet it actually is a hearing test. The words are presented visually but also auditorily at levels above and below the voluntary SRT. Moreover, the words are nearly impossible to distinguish just through vision because they are homophenous, that is, other words look exactly the same (e.g., cab, cap). The patient watches the tester (through the booth window) say the test words, while the words are simultaneously delivered through earphones. If the signal level is below the admitted threshold and the score is very low, the hearing loss is genuine. However, if the score is elevated, the hearing loss is false because the person must be benefiting from the auditory input. The point where the person shifts between an elevated score and a low score is very near the true SRT (Hamill, Karasick-Rush, & Segal, 1998; Weiss, 1971). A list of 20 words takes about a minute to administer, and it is not uncommon to administer several lists. The virtues of the Falconer test are its simplicity, the fact that no special equipment is required, its applicability to one- or two-ear FEHL, and its ability to predict threshold. Nonetheless, "lipreading" tests have hardly received mention in the literature.

Summary

This chapter covers behavioral tests designed specifically for FEHL. The Stenger tests rest on the principle that, when identical sounds are directed simultaneously to each ear, a person notices the sound only in the ear where it is louder. Whether using the tone or speech version, the Stenger test is most applicable when there is at least a 40-dB difference between ears in admitted thresholds. Signals are presented below the poor-ear threshold and above the good-ear threshold usually by 10 dB. If the poor-ear threshold is genuine or has an overlay of no more than 10 dB, the patient will notice the sound in the good ear and respond, which is a negative Stenger. If the hearing loss in the poor ear has a substantial false portion of at least 40 dB, the patient will hear the sound in that ear but not acknowledge it, which is a positive Stenger. A false component in the good ear makes it much less likely that a sizable false component in the poor ear will be found. Organic hearing losses generally do not play a role.

The Stenger test can provide a reasonable estimate of true threshold. To calculate it, the sensation level in the good ear is subtracted from the minimum contralateral interference level in the poor ear to compensate for the level above threshold in the good ear. Under good conditions the Stenger test is nearly unbeatable.

Story tests present different information to either ear or to both. Some of the information is presented below the volunteered threshold. The person retells the story or answers questions about it. If the person includes information that was supposedly inaudible, one has strong evidence that the loss is nonexistent or less than portrayed. The Falconer "lipreading" test presents words that, through vision alone, are not distinguishable from other similar words because they look alike on the lips. But when the words are presented along with their sound, word identification is very much easier. The sound level is kept below supposed threshold. If the score is high, it must be because the person was aided by the auditory cues in addition to the visual cues, which is evidence that hearing is better than alleged.

Now that the array of behavioral measures has been covered, it is time to turn to objective measures for FEHL.

Chapter 8

OBJECTIVE MEASURES OF AUDITORY FUNCTION

James W. Hall III
James E. Peck

Especially considering test efficiency, the results support the inclusion of DPOAE analysis in the diagnostic management of the suspect-nonorganic patient.

—Durrant, Kesterson, and Kamerer, 1997, p. 361

Normal thresholds by ABR do not constitute proof of pseudohypacusis, nor do they guarantee normal hearing. The ABR simply indicates the integrity of the system through the brain stem. This objective measure of system integrity, however, can be a powerful tool in the assessment of pseudohypacusis, especially when used in conjunction with other tests.

—Sanders and Lazenby, 1983, p. 297

Introduction

The two preceding chapters provided a detailed look at behavioral tests for FEHL. This chapter discusses objective measures as they relate to FEHL. Objective measures of auditory function are categorized as either electroacoustic or electrophysiologic procedures. Otoacoustic emissions (OAEs) and aural immittance measures (tympanometry and acoustic reflexes) fall into the electroacoustic category, whereas electrophysiologic procedures include all of the auditory evoked responses. For a detailed recent review of these techniques in the identification and diagnosis of auditory dysfunction in children and adults, the reader is referred to *Objective Assessment of Hearing* (Hall & Swanepoel, 2010).

Objective procedures depend on instrumentation to record some physiologic reaction to sound instead of a patient's conscious response. However, some clinicians have argued that the term "objective" is inappropriate because the electroacoustic or electrophysiologic response must still be analyzed and interpreted subjectively by the person conducting the procedure. Yet, formal investigation has shown remarkable interjudge correlation in the analysis of electroacoustic and electrophysiologic findings for patients with various auditory pathologies. Also, for some physiological responses, computer algorithms permit automated analysis, thereby eliminating any opportunity for subjective errors. Indeed, studies comparing automated analysis with visual inspection analyses have confirmed no important differences. Table 8–1 lists the strengths and weaknesses of electroacoustic and electrophysiologic auditory measure in the evaluation of pseudohypacusis.

Immittance Measures

Background and Rationale

Aural immittance measurements are quick and technically simple, and can be recorded in persons of all ages without regard to such listener variables as attention, motivation, developmental level, or cognitive status, provided there is passive cooperation. They also are handy in that tympanometry and acoustic reflex testing often are included in an audiologic evaluation, as opposed to other physiologic measures (Mehta 2003). Acoustic reflex thresholds for different stimuli have been useful for objectively estimating degree of hearing loss in patients who cannot or will not yield valid pure-tone findings. However, normal middle ear function must first be confirmed through tympanometry to ensure that acoustic reflex findings have credibility.

The normal range of the acoustic reflex threshold (ART) elicited by pure tones is 70 to 100 dB HL with an average of 85 dB. Cochlear hearing impairments ranging from none to a 60 dB have little effect on the ART. As hearing losses exceed 60 dB, the likelihood of finding a reflex threshold in the normal range decreases and the probability of an absent reflex increases. As a result, if a reflex threshold is only 60 dB or less above the behavioral hearing

Table 8–1. Summary of the General Clinical Strengths and Weaknesses of Electroacoustic and Electrophysiologic Auditory Measures in the Evaluation of False and Exaggerated Hearing Loss

Strengths

- Do not require a behavioral response from the patient
- Results are not influenced by motivation
- Results are not influenced by cognitive status
- Results generally are not influenced by state of arousal
- Measurements can be made with patient sedated or anesthetized
- Results are not influenced by the patient's native language
- Patient is not required to follow detailed verbal instructions
- Results are not influenced by motor status
- Measures provide information on multiple regions of the auditory system from the middle ear to the cerebral cortex
- Generally have high degree of sensitivity to auditory dysfunction
- Generally provide site specific information on auditory dysfunction
- Reasonable test time

Weaknesses

- Do not measure "hearing"
- Abnormal finding does not invariably indicate hearing loss
- Single measure generally provides limited information on hearing status
- Little or no information obtained about speech perception or understanding

threshold, one has strong evidence of a cochlear lesion. However, if the difference between the ART and the voluntary hearing threshold becomes very small, namely, only 10 dB or less, in all probability the hearing threshold is exaggerated. Certainly, if an acoustic reflex is found at or below the voluntary hearing threshold, that threshold is invalid.

Research Evidence and Clinical Reports

Gelfand, Schwander, and Silman (1990) determined the 10th percentile cutoff of the activating level for the ART (i.e., the low end of triggering the reflex). For hearing losses 65 through 80 dB HL, whether at 500, 1000, or 2000 Hz, the 10th percentile of the ART was 20 dB above hearing threshold (e.g., for a 75-dB loss, the 10th percentile ART was 95 dB). For a loss of 85 dB, the 10th percentile was 15 dB above audibility. It seems reasonable that, if the difference between the ART and voluntary hearing threshold is below the 10th percentile, there is ample reason to doubt the hearing threshold. Then, the clinician could take further steps to check the patient's response validity. In summary, the ART for pure tones is useful, provided there is hearing loss greater than 60 dB; for hearing loss less than 60 dB, the presence or absence of the ART has no value in identifying FEHL.

In the 1970s, acoustic reflex measurements were adapted to predict hearing sensitivity in infants (sensitivity prediction from the acoustic reflex or the SPAR). The underlying principle is that in normal ears the acoustic reflex threshold is correlated with stimulus bandwidth: the wider the bandwidth, the lower the ART, and the narrower the bandwidth, the higher the ART (Jerger, Burney, Mauldin, & Crump, 1974). The key for predicting degree of hearing loss is that sensorineural hearing impairments raise the ART more for broadband noises than for tones. Put another way, as hearing gets worse, the difference between the reflex thresholds for broadband noises and for tones becomes smaller. Typical ART differences for four categories of hearing are: normal hearing 20 dB, mild and moderate sensorineural hearing impairments 10 to 19 dB, severe losses less than 10 dB, and profound losses no reflex (Jerger et al., 1974; Margolis, 1993). Overall, predictive power is fairly good but hardly exact, and there is a significant false-positive rate. Still, the ART can identify losses above 30 dB 90% of the time (Margolis, 1993). Gelfand and Silman (1985) cautioned about predicting hearing loss from the acoustic reflex when FEHL is the concern because of the precipitously sloping audiometric patterns often found among patients with exaggerations.

SPAR techniques did not gain wide acceptance, probably because of the physiologic variations in normal hearing individuals and loudness recruitment in hearing-impaired persons (Psarommatis et al., 2009). Also, because of greater effectiveness, auditory brainstem response testing became the method of choice for evaluating infant hearing, which had been the purpose of SPAR. Nevertheless, the SPAR is one more tool to check for and roughly estimate hearing level in questions of false or exaggerated hearing loss.

Otoacoustic Emissions

Background and Rationale

The otoacoustic emission is a pressure wave generated by the motility of the outer hair cells of the cochlea. In OAE measurement, a probe introduces into the outer ear canal a sound that is transmitted through the middle ear mechanism to the cochlea, where it activates the outer hair cells. In response, the outer hair cells contract and expand rapidly generating a signal—the otoacoustic emission—which flows in reverse direction from the cochlea through the middle ear to the external ear canal. The probe has a sensitive, miniature microphone, which detects the evoked OAE sound in the external ear canal.

The noise level ("floor") during OAE measurement needs to be no greater than the upper limit for noise in normative data. To be considered normal, an OAE must not only be detectable above the noise floor, but also have an amplitude reaching an appropriate normative range. Thus, an OAE can be present by exceeding the noise floor by 6 dB or more but abnormal by being below the lower limit of normal absolute amplitude.

The likelihood of registering either normal OAEs or low-amplitude OAEs (activity above the noise floor but below normal amplitude) correlates with the extent of cochlear damage. This relationship between hearing level and OAEs is fundamental to detecting or confirming FEHL. As hearing thresholds worsen, even within the range of "normal hearing sensitivity" (0 to 20 dB HL), the amplitude of OAEs decreases. In persons with mild sensory hearing loss (20 to 30 dB HL), OAEs may be present but they have unequivocally low amplitude.

Sensory (outer hair cell) hearing loss is not compatible with normal OAE results. Normal-amplitude OAEs at all frequencies means that pure-tone and speech thresholds should be in the normal range of 0 to 15 dB HL, and certainly no worse than 20 dB HL. Otherwise, any degree of sensory hearing loss suggested by behavioral testing is dubious. The discrepancy warrants consideration of technical problems (earphone or earphone placement), nonpathologic subject factors (patient not understanding the behavioral task), or pathologic factors (isolated inner hair cell dysfunction or neural pathology). Early detection of FEHL is enhanced when normal OAEs are documented before performing pure-tone and speech audiometry, because a hearing loss by behavioral tests would then be immediately suspect.

The reverse pattern of findings, namely, abnormal OAEs in a patient with entirely normal pure tone thresholds (hearing levels 15 dB or better), occurs infrequently. Assuming normal middle ear function, there may be a technical problem, inner hair cell damage, or a neural disorder. Pertinent patient factors may be deduced from the case history. Because behavioral hearing thresholds are normal, a finding of abnormal OAEs is not relevant to FEHL.

The rationale for recording OAEs in the assessment of FEHL, and some limitations of OAEs, are summarized in Table 8-2. Although the advantages are compelling, the constraints also must be pointed out. OAEs have no diagnostic value in patients with even mild dysfunction of the middle ear. Also, OAEs may be absent or markedly abnormal when a false overlay is superimposed on a real cochlear (outer hair cell) hearing loss. OAE testing is a valuable component of the diagnostic battery, but it is by no means a test of hearing. Finally, OAE measurements always must be interpreted in combination with other auditory tests.

Table 8–2. General Advantages and Disadvantages of OAEs in Identification and Diagnosis of FEHL

Advantages

- Highly sensitive to cochlear (outer hair cell) function
- Site specific (to outer hair cells)
- Do not require behavioral participation or response; only being still
- Ear specific
- Highly frequency specific (multiple interoctave frequencies)
- Sound-treated environment not required for measurement
- Brief measurement time (<30 seconds for screening protocols)
- Portable (handheld) devices
- Relatively inexpensive
- Available in most clinical facilities
- Multiple billing codes for screening versus diagnostic tests

Disadvantages

- Susceptible to the effects of ambient and physiologic noise
- Affected greatly by middle ear status. OAEs generally not present in patients with middle ear dysfunction (e.g., otitis media)
- Evaluate cochlear integrity only for outer hair cells (not inner hair cells)
- May be abnormally reduced in amplitude or not detected despite normal audiogram
- Not detected with hearing loss >40 dB HL
- Provide no information on the degree of hearing loss
- Not a measure of neural or CNS auditory function
- Not a test of hearing

Research Evidence and Clinical Reports

Musiek, Bornstein, and Rintelmann (1995) demonstrated the efficacy of OAE testing in persons with false hearing loss. Five female cases of FEHL were tested via transient evoked otoacoustic emissions (TEOAEs). All had normal TEOAEs, which were in accord with ABR and middle latency evoked potentials. TEOAEs can cross-check the validity of subjective audiologic thresholds.

Durrant, Kesterson, and Kamerer (1997) examined the utility of distortion-product otoacoustic emissions (DPOAEs) in the assessment of patients suspected of FEHL. The majority of the 30 cases were confirmed as having invalid voluntary results through the aid of DPOAE testing. Some of those patients had false hearing loss and some had exaggerated organic hearing loss. The authors advocated including distortion product OAE analysis when evaluating patients suspected of presenting FEHL.

Saravanappa, Mepham, and Bowdler (2005) reported that their practice shifted to relying more on OAE testing and less on speech audiometry for identifying FEHL in children. In most cases, discovering invalid results can be accomplished through conventional audiologic procedures, especially with children. However, for more difficult cases, OAE testing is superior to behavioral measures because it is objective and bypasses the human element. Also, it is simpler, more convenient, and less expensive than ABR. They added that explaining the results of the objective OAE testing to children prompted improved voluntary thresholds.

Liberal use of OAE analysis can reduce the rates of late identified and undiagnosed FEHL and the resultant mismanagement. Delayed or missed diagnosis can have serious consequences, including needless diagnostic procedures, erroneous steroid treatment, unwarranted exploratory tympanotomies, unnecessary cost, as well as avoidable prolongation of suffering related to some psychosocial problem. Holenweg and Kompis's (2010) 40 patients with FEHL eventually were found to have normal or near-normal findings on OAE and/or ABR testing. Two children and seven adults had been fitted with hearing aids at a different clinic. A major reason for missing the diagnosis, according to Hiraumi et al. (2007) is clinicians simply failing to keep FEHL in mind. Matters are made worse by a unilateral sudden hearing loss or by an accompanying moderate to profound organic hearing loss. Hiraumi et al. (2007) reviewed 31 patients presenting FEHL. A total of 14 patients received unwarranted treatment before the diagnosis of FEHL was reached. Eight patients were treated with steroids. Six of those had presented with unilateral sudden hearing loss, and the other two patients had accompanying bilateral organic hearing losses. They advised using a physiologic test as soon as there is a question about validity in order to reduce the number of missed diagnoses.

Sakashita, Shibata, Yamane, and Hashimoto (2004) reported two examples of an organic hearing loss making it more difficult to find true hearing thresholds in exaggerated hearing loss. In both cases the pure-tone and speech audiometric results in one ear were not compatible. In the first case, an ABR threshold of 20 dB nHL argued for probable normal hearing sensitivity. However, subsequent OAE testing revealed moderate to severe hearing loss at low and mid frequencies up to1500 Hz. In the other case, ABR evaluation indicated a mild hearing loss in the suspect ear. OAEs were not normal above 3000 Hz, supporting a moderate to severe high-frequency hearing loss. Follow-up pure-tone audiograms of both patients ultimately agreed with the objective results. Because OAE testing gives frequency-specific information about cochlear function, it can be helpful in identifying those regions of the portrayed hearing loss that are genuine.

FEHL can easily be overlooked when someone presents with what seems to be an idiopathic sudden-onset sensorineural hearing loss (ISSHL). This is especially so when the complaint is only about one ear, because a patient's good ability to understand speech does not draw attention, given the one normal ear. Morita, Suzuki, and Iizuka (2010) described findings for 47 children, who at first were thought to have ISSHL but ultimately were found to have FEHL. Distortion product otoacoustic emissions (DPOAEs) were present in the 41 children who had normal middle ear function (the remaining 6 had ventilation tubes). Similarly, Oishi and colleagues (Oishi et al., 2009) encountered six adult females who appeared to have ISSHL in one ear. The patients received steroid treatment before OAE and ABR testing confirmed that the hearing losses were false. Alleged sudden hearing losses are particularly problematic because good medical care of apparent ISSHL demands immediate steroid therapy. In three of their six cases, ABR and OAE results provided the first evidence that these patients might have FEHL rather than

ISSHL. Finally, in the Psarommatis et al. (2009) series, 54% of the children with ISSHL were eventually diagnosed with FEHL. Normal OAEs were recorded for 45 of the 52 ears; the other 7 ears had a middle ear problem.

Because of its speed and objectivity, OAE testing is invaluable in complaints of ISSHL for ruling out false hearing loss. OAEs should be evaluated as soon as possible in all cases of hearing loss that supposedly come on quickly. Correct diagnosis avoids improper, expensive, and potentially dangerous treatment. ABR is highly effective but too time-consuming to use with each case, and acoustic reflex testing is useful but is not nearly as sensitive as OAE assessment.

Balatsouras and colleagues (2003) demonstrated the benefits of including tympanometry and OAE measures on 72 patients with suspected FEHL. One group (control) underwent an initial and a repeat speech and pure-tone threshold test as well as an ABR evaluation. The second group (treatment) had the same conventional and ABR testing but was also tested by TEOAEs and tympanometry. Both groups displayed better pure-tone thresholds on the repeat audiometry. The exaggeration level identified in the treatment group was larger than that found in the control, 35 dB to 11 dB. Also, there was no difference between the repeat pure-tone average and the mean click ABR threshold for the treatment group, but the pure-tone average was significantly poorer than the click ABR thresholds for the control group. Informing a patient about the normal objective test results may lead to valid behavioral estimations of thresholds.

Despite their enthusiasm for electrophysiologic procedures, Balatsouras et al. (2003) reiterated that these procedures are not behavioral tests of hearing. Every effort should be made to obtain accurate behavioral thresholds. Only when behavioral means are unsuccessful should electrophysiologic tests be performed. Qiu et al. (1998) had a similar point of view. OAEs were the most rapid, economical, and objective method of confirming the diagnosis of hearing loss in 78% of their cases. Only 15% of their subjects required ABR evaluation to substantiate the diagnosis of genuine hearing loss. In their opinion, OAEs and ABRs are needed for confirmation of peripheral auditory sensitivity in "more complex cases."

Auditory Brainstem Response (ABR) and Auditory Steady State Response (ASSR)

Background and Rationale

All the tests of evoked potentials are accomplished by delivering various sounds to patients and recording the bioelectrical voltages or potentials with electrodes affixed to the skin on the head. To elicit the ABR, the signals are clicks or tone bursts. The signals used to elicit the ASSR are rapidly varying sinusoidal tones. Finally, to test the cortical response, the signals include tones, complex sounds, and speech. The ABR and the ASSR can be reliably recorded in persons who are sedated or lightly anesthetized (although this is rarely necessary with regard to FEHL), but cortical responses require a state of quiet alertness.

ABR applications in FEHL are primarily to verify behavioral results and to estimate auditory thresholds when behavioral results are invalid. Secondary application is neurodiagnosis of any retrocochlear and brainstem auditory dysfunction. The click ABR is less useful when patients have a probability of a true noise-induced high-frequency hearing loss, which usually is the case with adults (Qiu et al., 1998). Some of those cases have medicolegal aspects and require either confirmation or credible quantitative values for discrete frequencies. By recording the brainstem response for tone bursts and systematically lowering the intensity level, it is possible to track the ABR down to the lowest level where it is reliably identifiable. The tone-burst ABR provides objective, frequency-specific information corresponding to hearing thresholds for frequencies from 500 Hz to 4000 Hz, especially when presented in notched noise (Stapells & Oates, 1997). Over 90% of ABR thresholds can be expected to be within 20 dB of behavioral thresholds, and the majority will be within 10 dB.

The ASSR is similar in most respects to the ABR except that it usually is elicited with modulated sinusoidal (pure-tone) stimuli rather than clicks or tone bursts. The signals are repeated rapidly with either amplitude or frequency modulation. The auditory signals vary at such a high rate as to cause overlapping nerve responses, essentially a "steady state" response to an ongoing stimulus. The bioelectric response generated in the brainstem follows the amplitude and frequency modulations of the stimulus spectrum. Rather than depending on latency, ASSR depends on phase in the spectral (frequency) domain. The evoked activity is automatically detected and analyzed by a predetermined algorithm, eliminating subjective interpretation. The ASSR can predict the audiogram at 500 to 4000 Hz. Finally, a significant advantage of the ASSR is that it can be evoked with intensity levels as high as 120 dB HL, permitting threshold estimation in severe-to-profound hearing loss; the ABR is usually not recordable when hearing loss exceeds 80 dB HL.

Research Evidence and Clinical Reports

Several articles attest to the value of ABR in FEHL (Lin & Staecker, 2006; Saravanappa et al., 2005). ABRs evoked with clicks and, especially, with frequency-specific tone bursts can provide an estimate of auditory thresholds in patients who do not volunteer valid pure-tone thresholds. A good example is Sanders and Lazenby (1983), who found normal or near-normal hearing by click-evoked ABR in four FEHL patients. Then, voluntary thresholds improved markedly, including in two patients who gave responses in the normal range. The behavioral results were commensurate with the ABR results.

De Koker (2004) studied the clinical value of ASSR in mine workers with genuine noise-induced hearing impairment, some of whom exaggerated their high-frequency hearing loss. In 81 cooperative subjects, the mean threshold estimates by ASSRs were within 10 dB of mean pure-tone thresholds, regardless of severity and age. In the 29 noncooperative workers, the ASSR and pure-tone thresholds differed by 61 dB. Hearing was successfully evaluated in 97% of this sample. De Koker concluded that the ASSR measure is a reliable and valid alternative to pure-tone testing in populations with noise-induced hearing loss, including uncooperative individuals.

Kariya, Fukushima, Kawasaki, Kataoka, and Nishizaki (2008) compared auditory steady-state response thresholds and standard pure-tone thresholds between patients with false hearing loss and patients with sensorineural hearing loss. Thresholds of 16 patients

(24 ears) with false hearing loss and 17 patients (24 ears) with sensorineural hearing loss were established at 500, 1000, 2000 and 4000 Hz. In the subjects with false loss, pure-tone audiometric thresholds and ASSR thresholds were significantly different, whereas in the subjects with sensorineural hearing loss, the thresholds did not differ significantly. ASSR testing may be particularly helpful at low frequencies.

Cortical Auditory Evoked Response

Background and Rationale

The cortical evoked response gives close estimates of true thresholds, ±10 dB, in the 500- to 4000-Hz range. Unlike shorter latency responses, the cortical or auditory late response (ALR) has the drawback of being diminished by the patient's lowered state of arousal due to sleep, sedation, and anesthesia. If the patient becomes sleepy or restless, the quality of recordings suffers, which may limit the number of frequencies tested to just two or three in each ear. That is enough to reveal FEHL and to form a good idea of a person's hearing sensitivity. Fortunately, these usually are not factors when the application is for the evaluation of FEHL. The cortical responses, when elicited by a complex speech signal, reflect a higher level of auditory processing. Indeed, the cortical auditory evoked responses are closer, in a sense, to a true hearing test than the brainstem auditory evoked responses.

Research Evidence and Clinical Reports

Thresholds of the cortical auditory evoked response typically approximate actual hearing levels within 10 dB in most patients (Hyde, 1997; Hyde, Matsumoto, Alberti, & Li, 1985; Lightfoot & Kennedy, 2006). As such, the evoked cortical response is well suited to determining frequency-specific hearing sensitivity in FEHL and medicolegal cases (Hyde, 1997).

Discussion and Concluding Remarks

The boon of having an array of objective test procedures is accompanied by the task of making a set of decisions. Should OAEs be tested on each new patient, even if behavioral results seem valid, in order to ensure that no degree of FEHL is overlooked? If confronted with an apparent FEHL, should all the objective tests be performed? Alternatively, should at least one objective measure be done? If so, which one? If OAE testing is chosen, is using a screening device sufficient? If the choice is an evoked potentials measure, should it be ABR? With tone bursts?

The great advantage of OAE analysis is much less time involvement, whereas the great advantage of EP procedures is the ability to obtain the equivalent of a four-frequency audiogram. Although OAE measurements are fast and dependable, a middle ear problem renders OAE testing useless. OAE testing is simpler and more convenient than EP testing and much less expensive. However, OAE testing is of no value in an exaggerator who truly has a hearing loss greater than 40 dB and wants the clinician to believe that hearing is even poorer than that. EP recordings would specify degree of genuine impairment in those cases, regardless of middle ear status or any organic disorder, but they cost more in time and money.

Perhaps a distinction should be made between diagnostic OAE testing and OAE screening. The latter is briefer and costs less. If screened OAEs are robust, the chances of a sensitivity loss greater than 40 dB HL are extremely slim (at least for the frequencies assessed). However, when faced with an apparent sensitivity loss across frequencies, which is the usual case in false hearing loss, a full diagnostic OAE analysis would be more informational, even if not helpful in estimating the degree of impairment.

If a clinician feels that not all but at least one objective test must be performed, given a question of FEHL, then selecting a test depends on the goal. When the goal is to verify behavioral results, recording OAEs would be in order. When the aim is to determine auditory sensitivity, then frequency-specific EP testing would be the procedure of choice.

One could make a good argument for using some objective measure on all patients. Often there is little or no reason to suspect FEHL. Also, the great majority of patients reporting hearing loss have a legitimate condition and respond reliably, so it is easy for clinicians to assume that the hearing loss presented is real. Furthermore, a good number of FEHLs present as a sudden hearing loss, which carries a sense of medical urgency to treat on the basis of "better safe than sorry." Another complicating factor in detecting a false component is an accompanying genuine hearing loss. All the above increase the likelihood that a FEHL will be missed.

There is another alternative that emphasizes flexibility and clinical judgment. The clinician can judge on a case-by-case basis, if there is cause for doubt, based on a sign or risk factor, which would call for an objective procedure. Conversely, one can assert that there are times when the indication of invalidity is so strong that using an objective measure to "confirm" it is superfluous. (Perhaps, the most powerful example is the unilateral hearing loss with no unmasked air-bone gap.) Many authors have argued that, when it is obvious the voluntary results are invalid, time would be better spent on using various behavioral approaches to seek valid voluntary results. Should those efforts prove fruitless, then a quantifying objective procedure would be essential.

Some authors advise routine use of EPs when FEHL is the issue. Others say that the EP measures, although exceedingly helpful, should be the last resort. The reason is the substantial investment in time to conduct objective threshold searches, especially at four frequency regions, and particularly in bilateral cases. Another consideration is cost. All objective tests, but especially the EPs, add cost beyond the basic audiologic evaluation.

Cost-Benefit Considerations

An issue related to deciding what tests to do is cross-checking, the principle of using at least two independent tests to verify a clinical outcome. The cross-check principle often is invoked in the literature on objective measures to give a higher degree of certainty to the behavioral results.

Some clinicians feel that OAEs should be tested on all new patients who claim a hearing loss. A clinical and financial argument can be made for doing so, but the main reasons may have more to do with the broader diagnostic value of OAEs than with just identifying FEHL. In any event, the presence of OAEs would rule out all but mild hearing losses. Also, by starting an evaluation on every new patient with OAE testing, FEHL will be deterred or detected sooner.

All of these considerations—confirming that nonsuspicious losses are valid, confirming that suspicious results are invalid, cross-checking, and testing every patient with an objective procedure—raise the question of the cost versus the benefit. Performing one or more procedures "just in case" adds significantly to the cost of hearing healthcare. Practical questions include, who is to bear the cost burden, and will insurance pay?

Let's consider the financial impact of routinely performing OAE analysis on every patient who reports a hearing loss. For sake of discussion, suppose that the charge for OAE testing is $50. Let's presume a 1% incidence of FEHL among the general clinic population, as suggested by the literature. One would have to test 100 patients at a cost of $50 each to detect one case of FEHL. That represents an additional health care outlay of $5,000 for one "hit!"

More realistically, we can suppose that the average clinician would detect a sizable percentage of invalid responders on the basis of behavioral audiometry. Thus, if the results of OAE testing indicated that 1 out of 100 persons was not responding validly, that one patient might well have been detected anyway. Let's suppose that the clinician would identify four out of five false responders. The clinician would have to measure OAEs on 500 patients to detect the one who would have escaped detection. Put another way, it means doing OAE testing on 499 patients, who either did not have the condition or would have been detected without the addition of OAEs, in order to catch one who otherwise who would have been missed. That cost would equal $25,000 per detection. An alternative is to pretest by OAE only select cases, such as those with a sudden or unexplained loss or progression of hearing loss, or those involved with litigation.

Resolution

There is no indisputable resolution to these questions. Whether to perform some or all objective tests on some or all patients on the first visit is a clinical decision. If a patient presents decreased hearing, OAEs might or might not support the behavioral results. If a genuine loss is supported, OAEs and ARTs together may shed light on the nature of the loss—sensory versus neural. EPs can help confirm or refute validity but they also can accurately estimate true thresholds for discrete frequencies. Ultimately, it is a matter of clinical judgment. The decisions should be made on the basis of the best information we have and in the best interest of the patient, including financial well-being.

Whatever one's views, there is no better way to guard against overlooking a FEHL than maintaining a degree of skepticism on every patient. The clinician must bear in mind that a complaint or presentation of hearing loss might not be true. This does not imply that most patients are untrustworthy or mentally ill, nor is the intent to make health care providers adversarial detectives. Rather, the rationale is to detect false or exaggerated losses as a matter of good care. It is not unfair to patients or disruptive to the clinician-patient relationship to maintain a certain level of suspicion, given that it is not in the patient's best interest to be misdiagnosed and undergo unnecessary and potentially harmful treatment. At the very least, clinicians must: (1) maintain an index of suspicion, (2) truly remain vigilant for signs and risk factors for FEHL, (3) use the variety of behavioral techniques that are available, and (4) employ objective measures, when obtaining valid behavioral results is difficult.

Final Thought

There is reason for concern about the "medicalization" of FEHL, particularly as portrayed in the literature on objective auditory measures, and especially in the medical and foreign journals. FEHL is described as the most common "etiology" of ISSHL. "Diagnosis" of FEHL and tests to "diagnose" it often are used as if FEHL were a medical disorder in contrast to diagnosing it as an audiologic situation. The word "find" is sometimes used as if finding the lack of valid results is finding something that exists. What is "found" is that behavioral test results are invalid, and (excepting organic components) there is no hearing loss. Related concerns are the emphasis on sophisticated instrumentation and elaborate procedures over behavioral procedures. As stated earlier, a behavioral approach usually is preferable, and the goal is valid behavioral responses. Finally, there is a dubious concept that FEHL can be "treated" audiometrically, that if one eventually obtains reliable-valid results, the "condition" has been "cured." If behavioral results end up valid, the condition has "disappeared." FEHL, by whatever name, is not a medical condition.

Whether or not a person truly has a hearing loss and to what degree are matters of importance, not only because of medical management, but also because of legal consequences. The genuineness of a hearing loss has tremendous implications for third-party payers, workers' compensation, invalid claims and undeserved financial awards, extra cost to businesses, or legal liability for clinicians. The next chapter covers those legal and forensic aspects of FEHL. It familiarizes the audiologist with the legal procedures and terminology one might encounter and provides information that will be helpful to the audiologist who may serve as a defendant, expert witness, or consultant.

Chapter 9

LEGAL-FORENSIC ASPECTS

Thomas Thunder
James E. Peck
William D. Domico

A competent witness with a valid point to make can create a poor impression without some understanding of courtroom demeanor, procedures, and strategy.

—Dobie, 2001, p. 5

Introduction

Audiologists may become involved in the legal system in a variety of ways. An audiologist could act as a consultant to provide an audiologic opinion on a forensic matter or serve as an expert witness. Audiologists could be called to testify or provide information about any of their patients, past or present. By being a treating professional, an audiologist could be named as a defendant in a lawsuit. All of these situations have strong relevance to false and exaggerated hearing loss. The purpose of this chapter is to provide the audiologist with an introduction to basic legal terms and concepts. Statutory and case law vary greatly among individual state and federal jurisdictions, and nothing contained herein is intended nor should it be considered as representing or conveying legal advice.

The term "forensic" conjures up images of deceased bodies, undoubtedly a result of the many popular television shows in which science is used to find the cause of death. In essence, forensic means "of or relating to matters of law" (Lat. *forensis*, of a forum, the public place of assembly in ancient Rome). Hence, "forensic audiology" is the application of the principles of audiology to legal issues or proceedings.

A substantial amount of forensic audiology involves litigation, that is, law suits. "Litigation" means a contest authorized by law in a court of justice to determine or enforce a right (Lat. *litigare* to dispute, carry on a suit). This is particularly true in cases where money is awarded, such as in a workers' compensation claim for damages for a hearing loss. However, forensic audiology has purposes other than litigation and courtroom testimony. For example, audiologic expertise can be applied in arbitration, technical guidance, consultation, or administrative hearings.

Language in Labels, Reports, and Testimony

Nowhere is the precise use of language more important than in the legal field. Careful expression, whether oral or written, is imperative. Audiologic notes and reports could become material evidence and, therefore, legal documents; thus, they should be written in a careful manner. A good report has kept many a clinician from potential liability.

A number of terms are best avoided. The use of the word "diagnosis" by audiologists has been controversial. Some staunchly defend their professional expertise and claim that, indeed, they do diagnose. Others, in and outside the field, disapprove of its use because of its wider, medical implications. Generally, a medical diagnosis connotes determining the nature and cause of a disease based on history, physical examination, and test results. One way to manage the controversy is to clarify that audiologists render an audiologic diagnosis, not a medical diagnosis. Another way (favored in this book) is to sidestep the issue altogether and label one's views as "audiologic impressions." Either way, you reduce the chances of an opposing attorney discrediting your status. To illustrate, suppose an audiologic evaluation shows a 50-dB hearing loss in the left ear with complete air-bone gap, normal tympanogram, and absent acoustic reflexes. The impression would be, "a moderate, conductive hearing loss in the left ear consistent with immobility of the stapes footplate as in otosclerosis."

Steer clear of terms that are outside the audiologic field. Two words that make the point are "malingering" and "unconscious." As seen in Chapter 1, Terminology, both refer to state of mind, and audiologists have no tools to bring such conditions to light. Moreover, in this context, malingering, is not a clinical matter for an expert witness to assert, but is a legal one for the court to decide (Main, 2003).

The most current or accepted terminology should be used, whether in clinical reports or in courtroom testimony. For example, the American Speech-Language-Hearing Association recommends "speech recognition" in place of "speech discrimination" or "speech reception." Informal, careless jargon, such as "bone scores," or "screening audiogram" (a contradiction in terms), is inappropriate. Using proper phraseology and adopting new terminology as it comes along demonstrate that the audiologist is well-informed and up to date.

A noteworthy example of the need for proper language and form is the report of an audiologic evaluation performed on a litigant. The report must be thorough. It should state the reason for the evaluation, relevant history, a description of the testing, and the audiologic impression based on all the above. The report should specify the equipment employed, earphones, speech audiometry materials, test procedures, quiet test environment, observations, anything out of the ordinary, and the audiometer's calibration status (Brady & Wilson, 2004).

Defendant

Audiologists are continuing to develop clinical practices as independent health care providers, the AuD degree being one of the more recent and salient indications. However, with increased autonomy, comes increased potential for legal liability. As such audiologists may find themselves introduced to the legal system by being named as a defendant in a lawsuit that alleges professional negligence (or malpractice). An audiologist can be sued, no matter how diligent, accurate, and ethical the person is. Thus, all audiologists must have professional liability insurance.

Should you become a defendant, your liability insurance company's attorney or representative will review your case, as reflected in what is often the most important and significant means of defense available and that is your documentation. Your records are legal documents, which, along with your statements and conversations with the patient, will be the basis on which your actions will be judged.

In any medical malpractice or professional negligence claim, the plaintiff will have the burden of proving each of these elements:

1. Duty, that a professional patient-client relationship existed;
2. Standard of Practice/Care, what an reasonable and ordinary practitioner would have done with this patient under similar circumstances;
3. A breach of this standard, that your care deviated from this recognized standard;
4. Injury, that this deviation, namely, your actions, directly caused harm; and
5. Legal cause, that the deviation was a legal cause of the injury.

Most, if not all states' statutes and case law require these elements be proved to a reasonable degree of medical certainty, or to be deemed more likely than not by "expert" proof. The plaintiff's word is not enough.

It is worth noting that not all acts of negligence result in injury or harm, and not all injury results from negligence.

Witness

Types of Witnesses

There are various types of witnesses. An *expert witness* is a person who possesses special knowledge, skill, training, or experience in a particular subject beyond that of the average person and is therefore qualified to provide testimony. The expert witness does not necessarily evaluate the litigant personally, but tenders opinions after becoming familiar with the facts and circumstances of the case through a review of the relevant material (Domico, 1993). The expert's opinions should be "based on a reasonable degree of audiologic certainty." In other words, the court is not asking for absolute certainty, but rather reasonable belief within one's professional judgment.

As a practical note here for clinicians, the process of potentially becoming an expert witness begins with the attorney conferring with the audiologist to review the case. (A person is not an expert witness until so designated by the court.) The attorney lays out the main issues with sufficient background so that the audiologist can decide whether or not to proceed. The audiologist may wish to think it over rather than commit at that interview. Regardless of whether the audiologist agrees to continue, it is proper for the clinician to inform the attorney whether the testimony would help or hinder the attorney's case (Brady & Wilson, 2004). If the audiologist agrees to be a potential expert witness, the audiologist and attorney should come to an agreement about the hourly fee. Compensation would cover the time devoted to reviewing the case, attending meetings, being deposed, and so forth, as well as expenses.

In contrast to an expert witness, a *lay witness* gives accounts based on their understanding or perceptions. A lay witness generally is limited to his or her personal observations. Audiologists can testify as a lay witness, but their testimony would not be from a professional standpoint. For example, if you saw a bank robbery across the street from your audiology office, you could be subpoenaed to testify about what you saw. In this case, you are a lay witness, but one who is also acting as a *material witness*, that is, having information that is potentially germane and significant. If you learned that a patient of yours was accused of a robbery but that patient was undergoing a hearing aid fitting in your office at the time, you could be called as an *alibi witness*. But, suppose you were called to testify against your will about a defendant charged with the bank robbery. Furthermore, suppose that you considered the person to be a highly honorable patient over the years. However, you did, indeed, see him leave your office and enter the bank at the time of the robbery. You would be considered an *adverse witness*. Finally, if you were called to testify in a child custody battle about how adept a mother was with her children when she brought them to your office, you would be a *character witness*.

Areas of Service

Areas of Service as a Witness

Audiologists are qualified to be experts in cases that involve hearing, noise, or audibility. The areas in which an audiologist could be of service include:

- worker compensation (relating to claims for noise-induced hearing impairment)
- administrative law (usually having to do with environmental noise issues)
- constitutional law (typically issues that involve the Occupational Safety and Health Administration or the Americans with Disabilities Act)
- tort law (personal injury, wrongful death, or product liability)
- criminal matters (e.g., a question of the audibility or intelligibility of certain events)
- professional negligence (commonly known as malpractice).

The compensation arena is perhaps the one most closely identified with forensic audiology. Some compensation plans are "scheduled," meaning that a dollar amount is set for various circumstances, such as degree of impairment, income, and years of work. Others are nonscheduled, which leaves the size of an award to a judge, jury, or other authority.

The largest scheme is the state workers' compensation system. Every state has a plan, but they vary in how they are constituted. For example, many states calculate hearing impairment according the American Medical Association formula for calculating percentage of hearing loss:

Percentage hearing loss for one ear:

1. Average the hearing threshold levels at 500, 1000, 2000, and 3000 Hz.
2. Subtract 25 dB.
3. Multiply by 1.5 to derive the percentage of hearing loss for the individual ear.

Percentage hearing loss for both ears:

1. Multiply the better ear's percentage of hearing loss ear by 5.
2. Add the better ear's percentage to the poor ear's percentage of loss.
3. Divide the sum by 6 to derive the binaural percentage of hearing loss.

Other states use different formulas; in some cases, which formula is used is left up to an examiner. Finally, if the claimant can prove gross negligence, some states provide for waiving the schedule, thereby allowing the aggrieved worker to seek compensation greater than on the schedule. Another large program, and one familiar to many audiologists, is the U.S. Department of Veterans' Affairs for veterans of military service.

Areas of Service Other Than as Witness

Beyond serving as a witness, audiologists are consulted to provide technical guidance or to educate the attorney in some audiologic matter. A lawyer might need an explanation of test results and a narrative report in everyday terms. Also, an audiologist's help might be sought to generate questions to ask the opposing side or to prepare responses to their likely questions.

An attorney may need an audiologist to evaluate a patient to help support the impressions regarding a case. The attorney may ask an audiologist to attend a deposition to help guide the line of questioning. An audiologist might be requested to observe another audiologist conduct an evaluation to confirm its veracity. Audiologists also may be asked to appear at a hearing or trial, not to offer an opinion, but to explain general audiologic principles or test protocols to the judge or jury. Because no opinion is involved, there would be no challenge to the audiologist's testimony.

As long as an audiologist is acting as a consultant and has not been named as an expert, then such work is covered by "*privilege*." That means the audiologist generally cannot be deposed or questioned by an opposing counsel (Sacks, 1995). At some point, your attorney may want you to express an opinion on the case. That requires your permission to disclose you as an expert witness and then to make this disclosure by a certain date as set by the judge. Without this disclosure, the audiologist would not be allowed to testify, except perhaps as a rebuttal witness. Although common in movies, surprise last-minute witnesses are nonexistent in trials that audiologists would serve in.

If in the early stage of your preparation you feel the evidence in the case is leading you in a direction different from what the attorney who hired you believes, you must so inform him as soon as possible. The attorney may then decide not to name you as an expert in the case to keep your information privileged.

To Qualify as a Witness

To allow the testimony of an audiologist, the court requires that:

1. the witness qualifies as an expert;
2. the field and methodology of the expert are reliable and valid;
3. the testimony will assist the jury in understanding the case or in deciding the issues.

Audiologists generally are deemed qualified to testify about matters within the profession's scope of practice, because they undergo specialized, graduate-level training in accredited schools. Also, an audiologist's knowledge of acoustics, hearing, hearing disorders, and auditory evaluation exceeds the common knowledge of ordinary people. However, whether an audiologist is granted the status of "expert witness" rests with the judge.

With regard to audiology as a field and the reliability and validity of our methods, audiologic principles and practices are based on an enormous volume of research and advances in technology. Precedent shows that audiology has been recognized as a valid field, such that audiologists have testified in numerous proceedings.

Finally, the judge must determine whether the testimony would aid the fact-finder in deciding a case. The fact-finder usually is the jury; if there is no jury, a judge is the fact-finder (a "bench trial"). The fact-finder decides if facts have been proven. For example, a judge likely would not allow a meteorologist to testify that it was raining on the night of an event in question when a simple weather report would suffice. Similarly, if there are already witnesses lined up to testify that they heard a certain event, such as an alarm, the judge may deem an audiologist unnecessary and disallow the testimony in the interest of moving the case along. On the other hand, the judge may be more flexible and allow the testimony anyway to reduce the chances of an appeal.

Once an audiologist has been qualified by the court, the judge often instructs the jury to regard the audiologist's opinion as fact. However, the judge also will instruct the jury to take into consideration the audiologist's level of qualifications when weighing that opinion.

Characteristics of a Good Expert Witness

The list of characteristics that make for a good expert witness could be lengthy. Here are some prime traits.

Objective. The witness's review of evidence is unbiased and conclusions are reached independently based on all available data. The court views an expert as a "friend of the court" and expects impartiality. Although advocacy is for lawyers, objectivity is for experts.

Professional. The witness presents as a trustworthy professional by appearance, dress, and demeanor. The manner is businesslike but cordial.

Articulate. The witness uses clear, well enunciated speech in an audible voice.

Sincere. The witness is genuine and authentic.

Amiable. The witness is pleasant and gracious.

Instructive. The witness can inform, explain, and express views clearly in a logical progression of points. The witness uses plain language in terms that the jurors can understand.

Confident. The witness is self-assured, poised, and assertive without being arrogant or pushy. By radiating confidence, credibility is added to one's testimony.

Prepared. The witness is familiar with the issues and facts involved, has studied all relevant audiologic information, and has reviewed documents prior to the proceeding.

Tips for Testimony

Audiologists are not accustomed to functioning in the legal arena. For most of us it is a strange and intimidating environment. Here are some tips for giving good testimony.

1. *Be truthful.* This is the best guiding principle for any witness giving a deposition or taking the stand.
2. *Listen carefully.* Listen to the entire question and to precisely what is being asked before replying.
3. *Answer only the question.* Stay within the scope of the question. Volunteering extra information could accidentally weaken your testimony.

4. *Take your time.* Think before answering each question. Even though an opposing attorney might rush you, there is no obligation to respond quickly. Witnesses who take their time are perceived as being conscientious and concerned about telling the truth.

5. *Don't guess at the answer.* If you don't know the answer, don't take a stab at it. Saying, "I don't know" may serve well. Other things one might say are, "I'm not sure about that," "I wish I could provide greater detail," or similar phrase. If you do not remember some piece of information, simply say so. You can always ask to refresh your knowledge by consulting your records.

6. *Ask for clarification.* Never attempt to answer a question you don't really understand. Since lawyers are outside their field when dealing with audiology, they might confuse terms and concepts and ask questions that may not make sense. It is always permissible to ask the interrogator to qualify, clarify, or rephrase a question. If the question seems convoluted, request that it be broken up into separate parts, so you can tackle them one at a time.

7. *Look at the jury.* Making eye contact with jurors as much as reasonably possible builds a personal bridge and makes them more likely to trust and believe you.

8. *Be cooperative.* Your obligation is to be helpful to the court. However, do not be forced into giving an inaccurate answer.

9. *Don't show irritation or impatience.* Witnesses who display hostility or annoyance lose credibility, and their emotions may interfere with their testimony. Usually, the examiner is not rude or bullying, in part because it is unlikely to win sympathy from the judge or jury.

10. *Relax.* Although not easy to do, you can lessen your anxiety by taking some deep breaths and reminding yourself that you are the expert in your field. Another way to help compose yourself is simply to ask the attorney to restate a question. This affords

you a momentary break. Also, before you take the stand, ask for water to be available, so you can pause for a sip.

Remaining calm and cool will go a long way toward being an effective and accurate witness. However, a shrewd attorney can tie a highly qualified witness in knots. The witness could feel that an attorney is distorting or needling, and an attorney might do so if it is deemed in their client's interest. It should not be taken personally, and losing your composure will render you less effective.

Legal Processes

There are several steps in adjudicating a legal issue, from the initiating complaint to the settlement or verdict. The audiologist may not be involved in all aspects of the process, but some background may make you, the potential participant, more aware of the workings and terminology of the legal system and thereby feel more comfortable navigating it.

Complaint

In civil cases, an issue starts with a complaint, a call for action brought within the legal system. The complaint will name the parties, set forth the legal elements and bases for the claim, state the allegations against the parties, list the claimed injuries resulting from the actions of the defendants, and specify the patient's demands for damages.

Forum

There are different forums for different jurisdictions and subject matter. If there is litigation or a lawsuit, the complaint would be in a judicial forum.

Jurisdiction

Claims must be filed in the proper jurisdiction. Certain courts are given the responsibility for specific types of claims, such as worker's compensation, a tax matter, or traffic court. Municipal or district courts normally hear misdemeanor crimes and civil (tort) matters of low dollar amounts. Circuit or superior courts handle felony crimes and civil matters of high dollar values. Finally, appellate courts review the work done at lower court levels, which ultimately can rise to the State Supreme Court (Rabinoff & Holmes, 1996).

Venue

Claims must also be filed in the proper venue, which relates to the geographic location of the court and where a particular action may be brought. In general, actions against parties must be brought in the venue where they live or do business.

Notification

Once the matter has been filed properly, notification is served on all parties. Notifications include the complaint and a time limit in which the defendant must respond. From this point, the rules of the court take control, and the case moves forward in a fairly predictable course.

Discovery

Discovery is a process used by an attorney to determine the facts and circumstances of the case to be tried before the court. There are a number of discovery tools available to an attorney. Each party requests relevant information and documents from the other side in an attempt to "discover" pertinent facts. Discovery devices include depositions, interrogatories, requests for admissions, document production requests, and requests for inspection. The process often starts with simple interrogatories, which are a written set of questions directed to the opposing party with a time frame to answer. Here are some other tools of discovery.

Document production requests are a call for documents that may be relevant to a case. This is the element of legal proceedings most often experienced by audiologists in the form of a subpoena. A *subpoena* is a legal written summons requiring a person to appear in court or present certain documents to the court at a specific time and place. For audiologists, the request normally pertains to a past or current patient, and the documents requested are usually audiograms, test sheets, reports, progress notes, and invoices. You must comply with a subpoena, as it represents a court order, and sanctions can be brought against you if you fail to do so. If you wonder if the information requested is confidential or protected in some manner, be sure to contact your own attorney for advice.

Examinations are calls to inspect the evidence or to evaluate a plaintiff. They often are referred to as IMEs or Independent Medical Examinations. When a claim comes to an insurance company, it almost always arranges for an IME. If the claim is related to hearing loss, the company typically consults their own database of audiologists to find a convenient location for the examination to take place. Getting on the database can be as simple as sending in your resume with a cover letter expressing your desire to be included on their referral list.

A deposition is an oral examination of parties and witnesses out of court in which a person gives testimony under oath. This tool is considered the most powerful form of discovery, because one can prepare for it and because it affords the opportunity to ask in-depth questions and to interact personally with the witnesses. Because all depositions are arranged beforehand, the audiologist will have time to prepare and to review any records.

If your attorney wishes to ensure that your opinions are placed into evidence, then the attorney will call for your deposition. Your attorney starts by establishing your qualifications and having you explain your tests or how you conducted your records review. Then you are asked to state your opinions in the case. The opposing counsel will then have the opportunity to ask questions. Your attorney will be present and is allowed to express objections. Your attorney also may interject questions calling for clarification.

Depositions are recorded by a stenographer, who generates a transcript and places it into the case record. You are allowed to review and correct the transcript by "requesting signature" at the very end. If you waive that signature, the transcript is finalized and made available for review by interested parties.

The discovery process is intended to be liberal under the rules of evidence to eliminate surprises at a trial and to encourage a settlement. This often means that attorneys seem to go on a "fishing expedition" (i.e., asking questions that seem irrelevant or tangential at best). Sometimes, they may catch a detail in your response that they can follow up on, which may help them in their settlement discussions or at trial. Each side is entitled to know what facts and evidence the other intends to present at trial. Thus, not only will an opposing attorney ask what you intend to testify about, that attorney may ask what you *do not* intend to testify about. By so doing, if you try later to give a certain opinion that was not included in your deposition, the attorney can object and the judge almost certainly will sustain the objection. This usually means the attorney wants to ensure that you, as an audiologist, will not be offering opinions about medical causation or treatment. This liberal policy in our system must be effective, because nearly 90% of cases are settled before trial (Feder, 2000).

In providing your testimony in a deposition (or at trial), it is permissible to rely on facts or data perceived by you or made known to you at or before the hearing. You need not have conducted your own test or personally collected the data. That means you can use another audiologist's findings, if you deem that audiologist qualified. You may also draw on self-reported patient histories, because obtaining history information is accepted practice in the course of our professional work. Finally, you can rely on the opinions of other experts in other fields as background material. You may, for example, avail yourself of an MRI report, indicating no suspicion of abnormalities of the auditory nerve or brainstem, in formulating your opinion on the prognosis with a hearing aid.

The Pretrial Phase

Before the trial, attorneys will prepare exhibits, demonstrations, and witnesses for trial. The preparation of a witness is important, because the attorney wants to rehearse the questions intended to be asked. This also is your opportunity to think about the questions an opposing attorney might ask.

Trial briefs for the judge are generated that lay out the facts sought to be proved and a summary of relevant law and cases. At this time, motions can be filed that request the judge to limit the scope of material to be covered by a witness. They also can call for a summary judgment or a directed verdict by the judge that, if granted, could stop the trial before it begins. Judges are reluctant to grant such motions and usually allow the trial to proceed in the normal manner. Once the motions have been dealt with, a pool of prospective jurors is questioned by the attorneys on both sides. This provides an opportunity for a lawyer to ask the court to exclude a witness, usually because of a possible bias. Jurors are then impaneled with alternates added as deemed necessary by the judge.

The Trial

The trial is the presentation of the case before a judge so that the jury can render a verdict. Many audiologists avoid working on legal cases because of the possibility of having to take the stand in court. In reality, having to appear at a trial is uncommon. According to the first author's unpublished survey of 442 cases that used forensic experts, 70% were resolved after the expert's initial report was submitted. This means that if your report is well prepared, there is a 7 out of 10 chance the case will be settled and go no further. In another 18% of the cases, a deposition of the expert was conducted but there was no trial. Only 12% of the time did the case actually go to trial. Even if a trial ensues, a case can be settled any time during the proceeding up until the verdict is given.

Trials start with opening arguments that set the tone and allow the jury to know the essence of each side's position. Both sides have the opportunity to present evidence and call witnesses. After your attorney asks you questions in the direct examination, the opposing side can ask questions in the cross-examination. Often, there is a redirect examination and a recross examination, a sequence that can be repeated more than once.

Rebuttal is an opportunity for either side to refute any aspect of the preceding testimony, including by argumentation or calling a witness. Because so much information is exchanged in depositions and reports, rebuttals in civil trials are not common.

Once the case presentations are completed, the court then gives each side an opportunity to make closing statements to summarize their case for the jury. Then, the jury begins its deliberation. Sometimes, the judge reminds the jury about burden of proof. Whereas, in criminal trials, the criterion for a guilty verdict is "beyond reasonable doubt," in civil trials, the criterion for a verdict is usually a "preponderance of evidence that the claim is more likely true than not." In some civil cases, the judge may create a higher standard by instructing the jury that the decision should be based on "clear and convincing evidence."

Summary

There is a reasonable possibility that, in the course of his or her career, an audiologist will interact with the legal system. The more common ways are through being a consultant, acting as an expert witness, or having records subpoenaed. Another less pleasant contact is as a defendant. This chapter provides an overview of the legal system as it pertains to audiology. It recommends careful use of language, as clinical records can become legal documents in litigation. This chapter lists several qualities of an effective witness. It also includes practical tips on how to act in the unlikely chance of having to take the stand. Finally, the chapter goes through the steps in litigation from the initiating complaint, through attorneys' accumulation of facts, to conclusion by a settlement or a trial verdict.

Chapter 10

PSYCHOSOCIAL CONSIDERATIONS

Addressing the complex factors that underpin any presentation of non-organic hearing loss (NOHL) is essential to that individual's proper management.

—Austen and Lynch, 2004, p. 449

Introduction

As mentioned in the preface, clinicians often consider false or exaggerated hearing loss an exasperating annoyance. They frequently regard FEHL cases as a distraction from serving more legitimate needs (Campbell, 1998). Yet, as we have seen, there is a significant prevalence of psychological problems among these patients, certainly among children, and they deserve compassionate care. This chapter explores psychosocial considerations that might relate to FEHL. Chapter 11, which follows, looks at management strategies.

Psychosocial Issues

Background

As the word says, psychosocial is a combination of psychological and social factors (Mosby's, 2006). More specifically, it is the combination of thoughts, feelings, and behaviors with social situations, relationships, and pressures (Corsini, 1999). Both psychological and social factors can contribute to the onset, course, and amelioration of a disorder (Campbell, 2004). All FEHL is a psychosocial phenomenon. Given the complexity of human nature, perhaps the concept of simulation behaviors should include the mind-body connection under the term "biopsychosocial." That description becomes even more logical when there is an organic "bio" injury involved, such as a genuine, coexisting hearing loss (Austen & Lynch, 2004; Main, 2003).

Prevalence

According to the National Institute of Mental Health (2008), in any given year about 26% of Americans (57 million) ages 18 and older have a diagnosable mental disorder. Nearly half have more than one mental disorder. Two of the largest categories are mood disorder (e.g., depression, bipolar disorder) and anxiety. Close to 10% of the U.S. adult population has a mood disorder, often accompanied by anxiety. Indeed, major depressive disorder is the leading cause of disability in the United States for the 15- to 44-year-old age group, affecting some 15 million Americans. Roughly 18% or 40 million American adults have an anxiety disorder (e.g., nervousness, panic disorder, post-traumatic stress disorder). Therefore, by statistical probability, some persons with FEHL will have some form of mental disability. Likewise, it is reasonable that a psychological burden would increase the chances of someone feigning a disorder.

Psychological and psychiatric problems also are fairly common in childhood and adolescence. Nineteen percent of youth have some psychiatric problem at some time (Kashani et al., 1987). For example, major depressive disorder strikes 1 to 2%, and 17% experience at least some symptoms of depression (Sood & Sood, 2000). Depression rises sharply in puberty beginning around age 10 (Doebbeling, 2000), and it rises faster in girls, becoming twice as common in females by late adolescence (Waslick, Kandel, & Kakouros, 2002).

Depression

Depression covers a range of degrees and disorders of low mood. The primary characteristics of major depressive disorder are sadness and loss of enjoyment in activities previously enjoyed. Additional common symptoms are: marked change in appetite/weight, difficulty concentrating, feeling hopeless and helpless, feelings of worthlessness, difficulty sleeping or oversleeping, low energy, and thoughts of death or suicide (American Psychiatric Association, 2000). In childhood, the major signs of depression are similar to those of FEHL, namely, somatic complaints and a decrease in school performance (Sood & Sood, 2000; Waslick et al., 2002). Hearing difficulty may be considered a somatic complaint, even if unvoiced, and most children with FEHL exhibit a drop in school grades. Childhood depression is less recognized because it may not present with sadness, but rather with the above two signs along with irritability, lack of energy, and behavioral problems. Other behavioral clues are: weight gain, hypersomnia, less social interaction, and illicit substance abuse (Sood & Sood, 2000; Waslick et al., 2002). Some precipitating factors of childhood depression include parental divorce, family discord, lack of emotional availability of parents, and death of a parent (Doebbeling, 2000). All these characteristics are quite prevalent among children and adolescents with FEHL. Hence, some of our patients, particularly children, with FEHL may well be suffering from unrecognized depression, and the consequences often are severe.

Maltreatment

Maltreatment includes abuse and neglect, and the two may overlap. Abuse and neglect can be physical and/or psychological (Hart, Brassard, Binggeli, & Davidson, 2002). Psychological maltreatment is embedded in all the other types and accounts for most of its trauma (Hart et al., 2002). Abuse of adults is quite broad, ranging from physical and sexual assault to domestic violence to stalking. Adult abuse and neglect often implies being vulnerable, as by age, infirmity, disability, incarceration, and so forth. Hence, compiling information on its prevalence or effects is very difficult. However, there is evidence that one in four vulnerable older persons is at risk of abuse, and probably only a small percentage of incidents are discovered (Cooper, Selwood, & Livingston, 2008). Although speculative, it is reasonable to suppose that maltreatment increases the chances of behaving in some maladaptive way, including presenting a false or exaggerated hearing loss.

Children, by nature, are vulnerable. The effects of child maltreatment include depression, reduced academic achievement, poorer social skills and relationships, aggression, low self-esteem, and risk of suicide (Erikson & Egeland, 2002; Kolko, 2002). In 1997, 2.3 million children in the United States were maltreated (Erikson & Egeland, 2002). A longitudinal study (Hussey, Chang, & Kotch, 2006) of a national sample of 10,800 children found the following experiences: 42% left at home unattended indicating possible neglect, 28% physical assault, 12% physical neglect, and 5% contact sexual abuse. It was estimated that from 2 to 4% of children in the United States are maltreated each year. All maltreatment predisposes children, both in the short and long term, to somatic complaints, depression, poor schoolwork, low self-esteem, substance abuse, unhealthy weight control behaviors, risky sexual behaviors, and suicide.

Gender

When compensation is the issue, most adults with FEHL are male. When compensation is not the issue, females may predominate. The male preponderance in compensation cases is probably due, not to inherent gender differences, but to socioeconomic factors, such as greater likelihood of vocational injuries, exposure to loud noise, and the economic pressures of the traditional breadwinner. Among children and young adults with FEHL, the literature consistently shows a 2:1 prevalence in favor of females. This predominance apparently crosses cultures: Greece 1.6:1 (Psarommatis et al., 2009), Japan 2.4:1 (Morita et al., 2010), Korea 2.5:1 (Ban & Jin, 2006), and Switzerland 1.7:1 (Holenweg & Kompis, 2010). The gender proportion of illness falsification of all kinds is 3:1 girls to boys, which is strikingly close to the gender ratio of factitious disorders among adults (Libow, 2003).

There is no clear explanation for the large number of females among children and young adults with FEHL. Perhaps, because girls with FEHL tend to be more introverted and boys tend to be more aggressive (Aplin & Rowson, 1986), females are more likely to internalize their feelings and express them with false symptoms. Depression might play a role in the gender difference. As noted above, the onset of puberty is accompanied by a disproportionate increased risk of depressive symptoms in girls.

Sexual abuse also rises sharply in puberty and occurs more often against females than males. Twenty to 25% of women and 5 to 15% of men have been victimized before adulthood (see Berliner & Elliott, 2002; Gordon & Schroeder, 1995). Rape happens to females nearly 4 to 1 over males and is notoriously underreported (National Center for Injury Prevention and Control, 2006). Furthermore, sexual violence starts early in life. More than half of rapes of women occur before the age of 18, and 22% occur before age 12. In 2003, 2 of 1000 children in the United States were confirmed as having experienced a sexual assault (National Center for Injury Prevention and Control, 2006). Approximately 20% of high school females have experienced physical or sexual abuse by a dating partner (Silverman, Raj, Mucci, & Hathaway, 2001). There is more relationship violence against females than males both before and during college (Forke, Myers, Catallozzi, & Schwarz, 2008). Before college, females are twice as likely as males to be recipients of emotional violence (27% vs. 13%) and of physical violence (18% vs. 9%) and three times as likely to be recipients of sexual violence (20% vs. 7%). The two main points here are that: (a) sexual abuse is much more likely to occur in childhood for both sexes, and (b) much more abuse happens to females in either time frame.

Apparently, at puberty girls differ from boys not just physiologically but in their social challenges. Their challenges may be more demanding than those of boys, and girls may react differently to them. The interaction of biology and social factors seems to form a complex situation that leads to a greater chance of depression in girls (DeRose, Wright, & Brooks-Gunn, 2006).

Suicide

Suicide deserves consideration because it is often linked to depression and maltreatment (Waslick et al., 2000). More than 90% of people who kill themselves have a diagnosable mental disorder, most commonly depression or a substance abuse disorder (National Institute of Mental Health, 2008). Depression is a leading risk factor for suicidal thoughts and completion in children and is also a prime symptom in suicidal children (Maris, Berman, Silverman, & Nesbit, 2000; Waslick et al., 2002). Thoughts of suicide, suicidal gestures (Sood & Sood, 2000), and completion rise greatly in adolescence (U.S. Dept of Commerce, 2004). Disturbingly, suicide tripled among adolescents in the United States between 1950 and 1980. Fortunately, the suicide rate for ages 10 to 19 fell from 6.2 per 100,000 in 1992 to 4.6 per 100,000 in 1996 (Centers for Disease Control and Prevention, 2004). Rates remained fairly stable in the years 1980 to 1995 and have plateaued at a somewhat lower rate since (U.S. National Center for Health Statistics, 2008).

Still, the increase with age is alarming. In 2006, the rate of suicide among 5- to 14-year-olds was 0.5 per 100,000 whereas among 15- to 24-year-olds, the rate was 9.9 per 100,000, nearly a 20-fold increase (U.S. Dept of Commerce, 2004). For those age groups, suicide rose from sixth to third place as a leading cause of death. Youth who consider or carry out suicide have low self-esteem, feel incapable of making an impact on their circumstances, have poor coping strategies, and are less able to consider alternatives (Maris et al., 2000). This does not mean that the typical child with FEHL is suicidal. However, some children in this author's caseload had expressed suicidal ideation.

This treatment of psychosocial issues is intended to show an interweaving pattern. Psychosocial disorders are quite common. People with FEHL might well have a psychosocial disorder. These disorders may stem from a variety of factors, including maltreatment. Maltreatment, especially of children, probably is more widespread than most readers would suppose. Maltreatment can lead to depression, poor self-concept, lower school grades, and unfounded somatic complaints (i.e., traits seen in children exhibiting FEHL). Depression and sexual abuse rise sharply in adolescence and are more prevalent among females than males, which is also true of FEHL. Depression, among other factors, can lead to the rare but catastrophic outcome of suicide.

Malingering, Factitious Disorder, and Conversion Disorder

These three conditions—malingering, factitious disorder, and conversion disorder—are the main psychological operations involved in health falsification. Here is how they are similar, how they are different, and how they can best be understood in relation to FEHL.

Malingering

The "malingering" label says that a person is trying to get something or get out of something dishonestly and knows it (i.e., an external locus of need and high intentionality). Viewed narrowly, malingering can be considered in simple terms as either present or absent. However, the issue often is more complicated (Main, 2003). The concept of malingering needs to be viewed in a broader way as part of a spectrum of exaggeration from slight to deliberate fraud (Main, 2003).

Although a valuable term, it should be used cautiously. As mentioned earlier in judicial matters, "malingering" is a legal, not a clinical, concept. Second, it has a negative connotation of dishonesty or weakness. The word may stick to a person and unjustly damage a reputation (Martin, 2009; Nemzer, 1996). Using similar labels, such as "functional," "faking," or "exaggerating" is ill advised for the same reasons. Even the word "uncooperative" is questionable because, for some patients, invalid responding is not intentional, and we cannot tell if a person's intention is to be less than cooperative (Gleason, 1958). The final caution is that "malingering" specifies deliberate intent, and clinicians cannot know what is in a person's mind. However, Austen and Lynch (2004) point out the value of the word and advocate keeping it because: (1) it is part of the widely used DSM nomenclature, and (2) it is unambiguous about degree of intent.

How bad or how frequent does a behavior have to be to constitute malingering (Raine, 2003)? Is malingering a matter of degree? Does it lie along a spectrum? The answers likely have to do with the magnitude, implications, and impact of the behavior (Raine, 2003). For example, claiming some ailment to get out of a minor household chore is trivial in comparison to obtaining a huge financial award after an accident. Also, the person to whom one misrepresents is a factor in its seriousness (e.g., to a stranger as opposed to a judge in a court of law).

Could malingering be a mental disorder? It is not included as a disorder in the DSM-IV but is listed as a condition requiring further attention. When measured against criteria of mental disorder, malingering does not fit well (Raine, 2003). Malingering is a form of dishonest behavior, sometimes extreme, but that does not necessarily constitute psychopathology. An alternative view is that all forms of simulation (malingering, factitious disorders, and compensation neurosis) are psychopathological syndromes. Hutchinson (2001) asserts that people do not simulate just for money; rather, their disorders involve attempts to resolve complex psychological and interpersonal issues. Specialists may disagree as to the extent that any simulating is a disorder, but they seem to allow that some simulators have more to their behavior than meets the eye (Rogers & Neumann, 2003; Sharpe, 2003). Currently, malingering is only a descriptive term for a specific sort of antisocial, possibly criminal, behavior and not of a mental disorder (Raine, 2003). Thus, the malingerer may be regarded as "bad, not mad" (Sharpe, 2003, p. 168).

To maintain some perspective, it is safe to say that we all have malingered. Indeed, probably all of us have at some time lied, cheated, or stolen, even if just to a trivial degree (Coles, 1993; Raine, 2003). Coles (1993) contends that everyone has intentionally presented some illness to escape an unpleasant situation or to get attention or sympathy (factitious behavior). Nevertheless, the great majority of people are decent, moral members of society. Thus, we must be cautious about being judgmental.

Seemingly, some clinicians feel quite confident that they "can tell" when someone is malingering. A danger in arriving at such a conclusion that way is the clinician's bias. One source of bias is the extent to which the clinician knows, likes, or identifies with the patient (Sharpe, 2003). Thus, categorizing someone as a malingerer may, at times, be a reflection of the attitude and reactions of the clinician (Sharpe, 2003).

Given the private nature of personal thoughts and motivations, it is difficult to know another's state of mind, and determining whether someone is malingering is hardly clear-cut (McCann, 1998; Nemzer, 1996). Certainly, auditory tests do not inform us as to a person's intentions and motivations. None of this is to say that people never fake a hearing loss with full awareness to get some external gain. We just cannot know, in the individual case, if they do so *purely* for external gain, or if there is some other motive unknown to us. The only sure way a clinician can know if a person is malingering is if the person admits it.

Factitious Disorder

Factitious disorder is a mental illness in which a person intentionally fabricates psychological symptoms or physical signs of a disorder for the benefits of taking on the "sick role" and not for external gains (internal locus, high intentionality). (A symptom is a person's subjective experience of a disorder, whereas a sign is an observable, objective condition.) The distinction, clinically, between malingering and factitious disorder can be ambiguous. The two are similar in that a false problem is knowingly presented. They difference is the nature of the resultant gains: external in malingering, and internal in factitious disorder. Deception can be established but the purpose might not be (Rogers & Neumann, 2003).

By "being sick," a person may receive emotional gains of nurturing, sympathy, attention, and the like. Sometimes, people will go to surprising lengths to appear sick or make themselves sick, despite substantial cost in money, health, or freedom (Miller, 2008). Laboratory results usually help establish the diagnosis. Factitious disorders are rare. The prevalence is unknown, but it is probably underdiagnosed (Sutherland & Rodin, 1990). These disorders have their onset between ages of 20 and 40 years, but usually in the mid-20s. Libow (2003) thinks most cases of factitious disorders in children do not fit the DSM-IV criteria and might better be termed "illness deception" or "illness falsification." It is typical for patients to be health care workers or to have some medical knowledge. It is unclear whether there is a sex predominance, although in some situations females have been found to outnumber males more than 2:1 (Krahn, Li, & O'Connor, 2003; Sutherland & Rodin, 1990). Factitious disorders tend to be long term and not easily treated (Krahn, Li, & O'Connor, 2003).

Even though, strictly speaking, factitious disorder is characterized by an internal locus of need, some people with the disorder might lie outside the region of purely internal gain to include some external gain. Similarly, even though factitious disorder is characterized by high intentionality, some sufferers might lie outside the region of strictly intentional toward lesser intent with correspondingly less awareness of what they are doing.

An example of the latter is the person who long ago realized that being "deaf" for psychological reasons meant that they got lots of help and didn't need to work. It is possible that people have engaged in a fallacious behavior for such a long time that it has become a habit. Habit is a conscious act, but one that a person might not be aware of all the time. People even may have forgotten, or never knew, why they engaged in the behavior. In the case of FEHL, they have adopted the untrue hearing loss for so long that they have even forgotten that they can hear (S. Austen, personal communication, May 31, 2010).

Conversion Disorder

In conversion disorder, the symptoms: (a) look like a disorder of voluntary motor or sensory function, suggestive of a neurologic or other medical condition, (b) cause significant distress or impairment, (c) cannot be explained medically, (d) are not intentionally produced, and (e) appear to be associated with psychological factors (internal locus, low intentionality). The distinguishing element between this and the two foregoing conditions is the quality of being unintentional. Conversion disorder may begin at any age but onset of symptoms is rare before age 10 and after 35 (Sadock & Sadock, 2008). In adults, conversion disorders are at least 2:1, and perhaps 10:1, more common in women than men. Among children, the female predominance is equally high or higher. Conversion disorders frequently are comorbid with major depressive and anxiety disorders. Regarding hearing, pure "psychogenic" (i.e., conversion-based) hearing loss is very unusual, although much depends on the exact definition of psychogenic (Coles, 2001). Most cases of childhood FEHL do not appear to represent a conversion disorder for two reasons: (1) most cases of childhood FEHL are identified rather easily (Mehta & Martindale, 2005), which is not characteristic of a conversion disorder, and (2) conversion disorders only begin to occur around age 10.

Scope and Interaction of the Deception Categories

Austen and Lynch (2004) assert that most people with FEHL do not fall at the extremes of either malingering or conversion disorder. Instead, they view them in a middle ground of factitious disorder, a sort of bridge between the traditional poles. The Austen-Lynch model is an enormous step forward in conceptualizing the thinking and behaviors of persons presenting FEHL.

Factitious disorder and conversion disorder have in common an internal locus of need. Factitious disorder and malingering have in common high intentionality. Thus, factitious disorder is comprised of both internal locus and high intent. However, Austen and Lynch consider persons with factitious disorder as having complex motivations and varying degrees of intention. Indeed, in their conceptualization, these three categories do not have rigid boundaries. Factitious disorder could extend to have some mix of internal and external need and also some blurring of degree of intention. That is why Austen and Lynch (2004) depict factitious disorder midway between malingering and conversion disorder, instead of where internal locus and high intentionality intersect.

Not only are the boundaries of these categories somewhat loose, the locus of need and the extent of conscious intentionality can change over time or vary with different episodes (Libow, 2003). Thus, a person might change diagnostic categories based on a change either in locus of need or in intentionality. For example, a conversion-based hearing loss could result in some external gain and then take on some element of malingering; conversely, an external gain does not preclude later meeting some psychological need and having some element of factitious disorder.

This nonpsychologist audiologist agrees strongly with Austen and Lynch that, when compensation is not involved, most children and many adults with FEHL are not malingering and do not have a conversion disorder. Their behavior seems more akin to factitious disorder, but often incorporating a blend of intentions, goals, and reinforcements. Moreover, it seems quite possible, if not probable, based on the literature that, even when compensation is involved, many individuals are not pure malingerers with no other troubling life situation that influences their thinking and behavior. Those individuals may know, deep down, that they hear better than they display, but they hardly are aware of why they misrepresent their hearing. They also may know that they are feeling negative emotions, but they do not make a direct connection.

The purpose of putting forth these ideas is not to suggest that audiologists should hazard a guess at a diagnosis. Instead, the purpose is to offer a framework from which clinicians can view the processes that quite possibly are in play in their patients. Happily, audiologists are not burdened with the responsibility of making psychological diagnoses. Our functions are to: (1) obtain the most accurate picture of a patient's hearing; (2) make the best recommendations; and (3) shed light, if we can, on the elements of intentionality and motivations (Austen & Lynch, 2004).

False Vision Complaints

Perhaps, it should not be surprising that there is a striking parallel to FEHL in the other special sensory system of vision. Suspicious or unfounded complaints about vision were mentioned in Chapter 4, Children. The number of similarities may tell us something about symptom choice and manifestations of psychological ill-health. Here are ways in which false and exaggerated vision problems are similar to those of hearing.

- lack of standard nomenclature (Griffiths & Eddyshaw, 2006)
- most of the literature has to do with testing
- history information is vital (Leavitt, 2006)
- often a legal question involved (Leavitt, 2006)

- seeking workers' compensation or disability (Leavitt, 2006)
- atypical reporting and behavior (Feldman, Eisendrath, & Tyerman, 2008), such as wearing sunglasses at examination (Bengtzen, Woodward, Lynn, Newman, & Biousse, 2008)
- extravagant claims about their difficulty and absurd claims for nonvisual sensory abilities (Feldman et al., 2008)
- inconsistencies between examinations (Leavitt, 2006)
- use of electrodiagnostic procedures helpful (Holder, Gale, Acheson, & Robson, 2009)
- psychological/psychiatric disturbances in the form of anxiety, depression, and attention deficit hyperactivity disorder in 27% of child patients (Taich, Crowe, Kosmorsky, & Traboulsi, 2004)
- significant home and school stress in 31% of children (Taich et al., 2004)
- 22% of children wanted glasses, girls over boys by three-to-one margin (Taich et al., 2004)
- predominance of females, at least among adults (3.7:1) (Griffiths & Eddyshaw, 2006)
- mental health intervention needed in many cases (Villegas & Ilsen, 2008)
- early detection helps end the false claim and avoids unnecessary treatment (Feldman et al., 2008).

Summary

Psychosocial problems, especially of mood and anxiety, are not uncommon. The same is true of various forms of maltreatment, such as sexual abuse. These influences predispose people to false disorders. False or exaggerated hearing loss is twice as common among female children and adolescents (if not also more prevalent among female adults), although reasons are unclear. There can be a web of interaction of multiple factors, such as low mood, severe anxiety, maltreatment, sexual abuse, and unfavorable circumstances, which increases the possibility of suicide.

The three categories of malingering, factitious disorder, and conversion disorder are differentiated on the bases of locus of need and intentionality. Even though malingering is not a psychological disorder per se, it is not considered healthy behavior. The boundaries delimiting these categories are not rigid. Factitious disorder and conversion disorder are relatively rare but are most prevalent among young adult females. A person can combine categories and even shift between them.

Whatever the origin, a nonexistent disorder, "is a symptom of something . . . [and] should never be disregarded or passed off as a temporary foible" (McCann, 1998, p. 175). In short, cases of FEHL should not be treated casually and dismissed quickly as clinical nuisances created by capable but uncooperative or dishonest individuals. The next chapter arms the clinician with a general framework as well as specific practical tactics to manage FEHL.

Chapter 11

MANAGEMENT: INTERVIEWING, COUNSELING, REFERRING

It cannot be overemphasized that proper audiological management of pseudohypacusic patients requires experience and skill not only in testing but also in counseling.

—Rintelmann and Schwan, 1999, p. 432

Introduction

Good advances have been made in identifying FEHL and determining true threshold, but management has not received the same interest or progressed as well (Mehta & Martindale, 2005). Perhaps that is due to low awareness of the psychological significance of FEHL and an undervaluation of the audiologist's role in managing FEHL (Austen & Lynch, 2004). This chapter reviews approaches to management. Any strategy that is adopted must address the fact that FEHL carries a significant risk of a psychosocial problem. In this chapter the audiologist will find ways to estimate that risk. The chapter also includes practical examples of how to handle sensitive issues in interviewing, counseling, and referring. Nothing here is a substitute for mental health care from a qualified professional nor are the contents meant as a guide for audiologists to act as professional mental health care providers. The intent is to help audiologists deal with the psychosocial aspects of FEHL.

Intervention and Management Approaches

What should audiologists do when they encounter a false or exaggerated hearing loss? One alternative—a dangerous one—is to do nothing. Even if the false hearing loss resolves during the evaluation, one still should check for signs of possible psychosocial difficulty. The problem does not disappear just because the "hearing loss" disappears. An opposite view is to refer all patients for further evaluation or to make a general statement that a psychological matter might be involved. The latter approach will result in overreferral or leave patients or parents at sea. A more efficient alternative is to assess the likelihood of psychosocial problems in order to best manage the situation.

The literature reflects a range of intervention philosophies from minimal to considerable. Some approaches consist of explanation, encouragement, and reassurance (Brockman & Hoversten, 1960). Others go further and include consultation with the schools, parents, and health care providers to help resolve any underlying psychosocial troubles. Bowdler and Rogers (1989) advised observation and supportive therapy. Veniar and Salston (1983) employed suggestion therapy by making an authoritative statement that hearing was improving and would be normal soon. Aplin and Rowson (1990) felt that the high prevalence of home or school problems was itself an argument for referring all children with FEHL for psychological evaluation. A psychologist or psychiatrist might be needed for severe or recalcitrant cases (Andaz et al., 1995; Pracy et al., 1996).

Despite differences in the various approaches, there tends to be general agreement on some points. Most writings on this subject are about children, but the ideas apply to any age. One principle is not to treat the person as hearing impaired. In the case of children, that would include no preferential seating in school. Treating someone as if they had a hearing loss would reinforce the idea that there is a hearing loss. Avoid discussing hearing altogether; if the subject comes up, reassure the person that the hearing was found to be quite good and is supposed to get better.

Views are divided on whether to attempt to identify the cause of FEHL in an individual. Brockman and Hoversten (1960) were wary about audiologists trying to identify the underlying problem. Veniar and Salston (1983) felt that questioning about a child's situation might "consolidate" the hearing loss. However, others have advocated trying to ascertain the psychological problems (Coles, 2001; Pracy et al., 1996). The various writings have great merit, as far as they go. A concern is for what was not said. Although authors encourage checking for possible psychosocial problems, they do not say how to go about it. Common advice is "intervention as needed," but there is a lack of direction about how to determine if it is needed.

Obtaining some sort of intervention or therapy is worthwhile. One stark example is the 8-year-old boy mentioned in Chapter 4, who endured a dreadful situation until it was changed by family therapy. "Excellent response" was how Lehrer et al. (1964) described the outcome of psychotherapy with a group of children who had FEHL. The therapy was largely supportive in nature and lasted from several weeks to 3 months (some therapy continuing at school). As school adjustment improved, the false hearing loss resolved.

Some cases of FEHL may resolve on their own, yet without intervention, resolution might require more time. With or without intervention, finding normal hearing on a return visit is not in itself an indicator of good mental health. Going by the results of a hearing evaluation makes the hearing test also something of a mental health test. Relinquishing a false hearing loss is a better sign than perpetuating it. However, a symptom could abate and disappear without the patient having become free of the causal problem, or the person could have shifted to a new false symptom. Furthermore, even if the "loss" (and underlying problem) resolves by itself later on, until then a person may be suffering needlessly. Intervention is not something to be avoided.

Interviewing

It is not the purpose of this section to cover all aspects of interviewing. Instead, the focus is on the sorts of questions to ask and how to ask them to decide whether there is need for referral.

This author has the impression that techniques of discussing delicate issues are not well taught in audiology programs, and that, in contrast to performing audiometric tests or fitting hearing instruments, such behaviors are not well modeled by mentors. Furthermore, there is a widespread myth that patients do not want to talk about psychological matters. In fact, they are as willing to discuss them as they are physical concerns, if they are asked (see Schneider & Levenson, 2008). The interview techniques for such matters are not complicated or difficult. However, they may not be familiar to audiologists and the subject matter may be sensitive, making use of these techniques intimidating. However, with practice, audiologists can incorporate these techniques into their routine and become more at ease in addressing personal issues. Here are some tactics.

Tactics

When there is enough reason to suspect FEHL, the clinician can begin by asking a few open-ended questions using tactful, nonthreatening language. The language is adjusted to whether the interview is with the patient or an accompanying person and whether the patient is a child or an adult. The conversations are quite similar, mainly modifying the style to be age appropriate.

To set the stage, this audiologist tells the person that obtaining the test results had been more difficult than usual. He says that every year he sees a handful of people who, at first, show hearing loss, but the tests come out normal. He continues that he often finds that those individuals have some "preoccupation" that is interfering with efficient listening. He may add that, when preoccupied enough with what is going on inside, we are less available for what's coming in from outside. He asks, "Might that apply to you?" If the person is noncommittal, a next tactic is to mention some typical symptoms—being uptight, having less fun, stomach trouble, and the like—and see if the patient can relate to them. The clinician can follow up by being more specific, asking in a comfortable and straightforward manner if there is anything troubling the person in three main areas: home, friends, and school or job. If the person indicates there is a difficulty, invite that person, "Would you like to tell me about it?"

If the responses to all of these questions are not suggestive of a psychosocial concern, the audiologist should stop. A clinician should not delve beyond what is helpful in deciding whether and what sort of further attention is advisable. Otherwise, the clinician should continue the interview. In the case of children 6 to 12 years of age, the caregiver can easily complete the Pediatric Symptom Checklist (described in Chapter 4). Also, the PSC can be a source of very good questions that the clinician can ask before or after the testing portion of the session.

Abuse

If something in the course of the visit suggests a cause for concern, give strong consideration to asking about the possibility of abuse, particularly sexual abuse. The very notion may be quite unsettling, frightening, and threatening to audiologists. However, recall two important facts from Chapter 10. First, sexual violence and abuse, especially against females and children, are disturbingly prevalent and often are implicated in psychosocial difficulties. Second, the results of abuse are serious and, at times, catastrophic. Even though it would be in the best interest of the patient, raising the subject may be awkward, and many abuse survivors are quite reluctant to reveal their sexual abuse to anyone (Read, McGregor, Coggan, & Thomas, 2006), so the situation goes unattended. If boys and girls do decide to disclose their abuse, they usually do not tell professionals but a friend of their own age, who is ill equipped to be helpful. Girls are even less likely than boys to disclose information about such experiences (Priebe & Svedin, 2008). Thus, health care professionals have a responsibility to inquire instead of waiting for a spontaneous disclosure (Read, McGregor, Coggan, & Thomas, 2006). A child who is being abused is not helped by the health care professional whose discomfort results in silence in this regard. Although patients are reluctant to talk about things of a sexual nature, it also might be the clinician who is reluctant to talk about them. Key to patient disclosure is having a good clinician-patient relationship (see Schneider & Levenson, 2008).

If the patient is a child or adolescent, questions about abuse—sexual or otherwise—can be posed as, "Does anyone hurt you, make you feel bad. Is someone not nice to you?" In talking to parents or adults, helpful phrases might be, "Is there anything in the area of inappropriate behavior that is a concern," or "I know a person who specializes in issues of abuse. Do you think there is any reason to consider getting that person involved?" If we as health care providers dodge asking about delicate matters when there is reason to ask, we might be failing the child.

It is crucial to realize that, apart from any concern about interviewing techniques, the mere suspicion of any sort of maltreatment probably carries a legal obligation to report it. In the case of children, states have laws that *require* licensed professionals to report suspected maltreatment. Informing one's employer, the referring party, or the primary care provider does not relieve the individual professional of the legal obligation of making one's own report. However, in the case of adults, a report might not be required, depending on the state. Indeed, for various legal reasons, a report may not even be allowed when the concern is sexual abuse of an adult. In all events, it would be wise to document the reasons for suspicion. State laws are fairly uniform, but if a reason for suspicion arose, the clinician would need to consult and follow the requirements of his or her state. These laws have provisions that protect the reporting professional (J. Gatewood, personal communication, August 3, 2010.)

Confidentiality

Any time a health care provider talks with a patient about powerful and sensitive issues, confidentiality should be assured but explained. A clinician could say something like this, "Everything you and I talk about will be confidential but I need to explain what this means here. Of course, I won't be telling our conversation to anyone who has no business knowing about it. But, as an audiologist, I am a member of a health care team. To help you, members of that team might share information with others of the health care team who have skills that could be beneficial to you. So you have confidentiality, not just with me but with anyone on the health care team. The only time that confidence might be broken is if we have strong reason to suspect you will harm yourself or somebody else, or if you give any information about any child 16 or under who is being abused. In these kinds of situations, we will break confidentiality in order to try to keep you and any other person safe" (S. Austen, personal communication, November 17, 2010).

Counseling

"Counseling" means advising or providing guidance and direction. However, as used in audiology, it often really means educating, such as explaining the audiogram or showing how to use a hearing aid. Many audiologists have not had coursework or training in personal adjustment counseling, that is, helping people deal with their communicative situation on an emotional level. They have not been shown how to differentiate between content messages (cognitive realm) and affective messages (feelings realm), and how to respond to each type, but those skills can be learned (English, Mendel, Rojeski, & Hornak, 1999). Much of "audiologic counseling" is informational, and the flow is mostly from audiologist to patient. In matters of FEHL, the contents should include a greater proportion of feelings and attitudes, and the flow should go more from patient to audiologist.

"Third Ear"

Effective interviewing and counseling involve listening with our "third ear" (English & Clark, 2003), that is, attending to more than the words themselves. It means listening "between the lines" to those feelings or hidden thoughts that may underlie what a person says. It requires a deeper level of listening to perceive how the speaker feels, attending to the patient's emotions, and truly acknowledging that we heard them. When this occurs, patients feel accepted and understood, and are more likely to express themselves and follow our recommendations. The requisite time may present a dilemma to the busy clinician, but one hopes that patient well-being is not compromised because of time or because the concern is not about an organic condition.

If the patient is a child, time should be spent just with parents and also just with the child. Afterward, time can be spent with both together. Time spent just with the child respects the child's individuality. By being alone with one and then the other, the clinician can be more frank, and the patient and the care providers can be freer to express themselves and ask questions. It may not always be possible to separate the child, but usually it is. To transition to conversing with the adult, one can tell the child, "You and I have already had a conversation; now I'd like to do the same with your parents." However, if having the child present is unavoidable, a later phone call to the adult may have to suffice.

When FEHL is involved, the patient/parent should be informed of the outcome of the evaluation, that is, whether or not hearing turned out to be normal and whether testing was unusual or incomplete. This is the point where counseling and interviewing merge. The clinician may ask about adjustment and behavior as mentioned above. At the end of that discussion, the clinician can bring up referring for further management.

Significant others need to understand that there must be no retribution or recriminations. Patients must not be confronted, blamed, or punished (Berger, 1965; Coles, 2001). In the case of children, explain to the care providers that the child is likely not being bad or naughty. Understandably, a parent could feel quite annoyed at a child wasting the time, incurring an expense, and giving them a hard time for no reason, and so forth. It can be helpful to frame the situation as the child is not giving us a hard time but is having a hard time.

If care providers become distressed that their child might be going through a difficult period, reassure them that the session is the start of good things. Set a positive tone that there is now perhaps less mystery and more understanding of the child's situation. The family has a better direction now in which to move. Thus, they can expect that things eventually will get better. In the rare instance of a patient wearing a hearing aid, but whose results show normal hearing (or no degree of impairment calling for a hearing aid), plan a program to wean the patient from hearing aid use.

The clinician should wrap up the session with the parents and child together. They should be left with the notion that hearing was "OK" and reassured that any hearing loss was fading and would disappear.

When talking to a patient/parent, we must resist the temptation to rush. Patients feel best about and are more likely to comply with clinicians who spend time with them. During a conversation, silence is not bad; often it is positive, as it allows reflection and also sends the signal that the patient is the priority and that the clinician is open to questions. By its nature, FEHL brings confusion and uncertainty, so be ready to say you don't know or are confused, too; this makes you an ally, a partner. Parents or companions often feel troubled or frustrated and want answers. "I wish I knew the answer" is a gentle way of saying there might not be an answer, or not yet anyway. Also, parents respond favorably to frankness and appreciate honesty.

"It's Not My Job"

A reaction from audiologists to many of these views on interviewing and counseling may be, "It's not my job." By listening with our "third ear," such a statement might mean, "I feel uncomfortable getting into such matters." Although that reticence is understandable, and to some extent wise, it should not deter us from all communication of a sensitive nature. As audiologists, we deal with (or should) issues that are not just about hearing but involve feelings. They require audiologists to be attuned to the emotional needs of the patients, to meet the patients where they are. It is futile to try to communicate when the patient is in the domain of affect and the clinician is in the domain of facts. If we overlook getting in touch with a patient's needs at a deeper level, we risk acting as technicians and not meeting our responsibility of making well-informed recommendations (Mehta & Martindale, 2005).

Conversely, audiologists must not assume the role of mental health professional. Overstepping our bounds has its own negative consequences. Yet, we can respond to a patient's feelings that are related to the audiologic situation. The degree to which each of us engages in such conversations will depend on our training, experience, interest, and aptitude. We need to remain mindful, however, of the needs of the patient and resist being frightened away by sensitive matters. Problems that are unrecognized or untreated can persist or lead to additional maladaptive behaviors.

Some may question whether certain of the goals and approaches discussed above lie outside audiology's scope of practice. The fact that much of the literature was authored by audiologists argues that this would be an overly narrow view, as would the various audiology books on counseling. There are issues that an audiologist might deal with that are not just about hearing but very much about feelings and adjustment. Examples are parents' grief over a child's newly found hearing loss, children and youth rejecting hearing aids out of embarrassment, a tinnitus sufferer distraught by the life-disturbing condition, or even identifying a conversion disorder in a person with chronic dizziness (Honaker, Gilbert, & Staab, 2010).

Follow-Up

Whether and when a person with FEHL should be brought back for an audiologic reevaluation is a challenging clinical judgment. If the matter is one of a reliable and accurate assessment for medicolegal purposes, obviously, the person must be seen again. In nonmedicolegal cases, it might be a matter of the audiologist's level of confidence. If there was enough uncertainty about a genuine hearing impairment, a follow-up visit would be in order. However, if the audiologist was confident that the patient's hearing was normal, even though the patient had performed invalidly much of the time, a repeat hearing test might not be wise.

Recall the guiding principle that nothing should be done to reinforce the patient's notion of having hearing impairment. A patient may wonder, "If my hearing is so good, how come they want me back for another test?" Supposing that, at the conclusion of the initial evaluation, hearing loss was not really in question but that the concern was a psychosocial one, a follow-up visit would be counterproductive. As long as the audiologist was confident that the patient had normal hearing in each ear, this writer feels that a follow-up visit, whether in a month or in a year, is contraindicated. A follow-up telephone call could serve fairly well to check on the psychosocial concerns and to decide if an appointment was advisable. Clinical judgment must weigh the benefits of not maintaining attention on hearing against whatever benefits there might be from a reevaluation.

Making a Referral

Central to being a health care provider is making clinical judgments. At some point, the clinician has to decide whether or not to refer. Having considered the patient's overall picture, the average clinician most probably has good ability to determine whether a referral is in order. One need not have evidence beyond a reasonable doubt, only reasonable suspicion of a problem, to initiate a referral.

Recall in the Peck (2002) report that a major issue was trying to estimate if a child was at risk of having a psychosocial disorder. Among the patients with FEHL that Peck encountered, 31 were children in the age range of the Pediatric Symptom Checklist, the screening test for psychosocial dysfunction. Of those 31 children, 23 (74%) scored positive for a disorder. The clinician's impression had been that 20 of those 23 children were at risk. Conversely, the PSC suggested that 8 children were not at risk, and the audiologist's clinical opinion coincided in 7 instances. Altogether, the clinical impression and the PSC score, as to whether a child was in jeopardy or not, agreed in 27 of 31 cases or 87% of the time. This should be quite heartening to audiologists, even though the above was a clinical report and not a scientific study. To the extent that the PSC is a valid and sensitive tool (sensitivity, 0.95; specificity, 0.68), the concurrence of the PSC outcomes and the audiologist's judgment suggests that audiologists probably have better judgment in such matters than they might think and can trust their instincts.

Once it has been determined that further attention is in order, the next step is to facilitate getting that care. If the patient has a primary care provider, it would be appropriate to suggest that the patient confer with that provider. If that is not the case, or if the patient/parent prefers to proceed directly to a mental health care provider, be ready to provide information. The clinician could maintain a list of mental health professionals with their locales, specific competencies, and contact information (Harvey, 2008). One could offer to call the provider either right then or later to help move the process along. If at all possible, call the patient/parent later to see if they followed through with making contact.

Examples of Techniques for Interviewing, Counseling, Referring

Here are some specific techniques for interviewing, counseling, and referring. Notice that the progression is from open-ended questions to narrower ones. They are applicable to patients and to parents. The list is not meant to be exhaustive. The sample wordings are merely illustrative; clinicians should use their own words.

1. Explain your reasons for concern, and then ask, *"What do you make of that?"*
2. Give a typical scenario of a person with FEHL, for example, a change in mood, a drop in grades, some unpleasantness in life, and ask; *"Might that apply to you/your child?"*
3. Open-ended questions increase flow of information, such as, *"How are things going?"*
4. If something negative is mentioned, follow with, *"Tell me about that."*
5. Move toward more focused items, such as:
   - changes in behavior or personality (brooding, acting younger, touchier)
   - somatic complaints, especially ones that are suspect or unsubstantiated, for example, headache or stomachache
   - increasingly withdrawn, wanting to be alone more
   - feeling sad, teary, hopeless, having less fun
   - recent separation of a loved one (death, divorce, separation, move)
   - less energetic.
6. Listen; promote safe, confidential environment.
7. Questions might be statements in disguise. For example, a mother saying, *"Do you think her father and me splitting up could be a factor?"* might mean, *"All this began about the time her father and I fought a lot and then separated. I think it really bothered her, and I feel guilty."* One possible way to respond is to reverse the question and say, *"I don't know. Do you have any thoughts on that?"*
8. Be nondirective and client centered. This style is unfamiliar to many audiologists because it differs from the standard clinician-centered model in which the authority figure does most of the

talking. Rather, it encourages patient expression by acceptant, nonjudgmental reflecting, rewording, clarifying, and repeating.

9. Repeating or rewording what someone says prompts more expression. For example, Parent: *"She gets in trouble at school."* Audiologist: *Hmm, so she gets in trouble at school."* Or, Parent: *"He fights all the time."* Audiologist: *"He does a lot of fighting?"*
10. One may need to lead the patient, such as saying *"What else?"* Or, *"You mentioned that a relative passed away. Was that a particularly difficult time for you/your child?"*
11. Asking or wondering is less threatening than telling. *"Do you think he feels a need for more attention?"* or *"I wonder if he's feeling that he doesn't get enough attention?"* versus *"It seems to me, he needs more attention."*
12. Continuation cues: *"Go on. Uh huh. Continue with what you were saying. Really?"*[1]
13. Reduce embarrassment with questions that imply normal: *"What with having to change schools and make new friends, I wonder if you would just rather stay home alone?"*[1]
14. Reduce threat by symptom expectation. To make the point, note the same wording as above except at the end: "*What with having to change schools and make new friends, I would think you would just rather stay home alone."*[1]
15. Reduce threat by showing the client not alone: "*I see people/kids like you every year and they feel bad about their marriage/school and have bad thoughts. Has that happened to you?"*[1]
16. Use exaggeration to suggest a frequency higher than expected, so the patient feels the behavior isn't so bad. *"Some kids cut school all the time. What about you?"*[1]
17. Reflect on what the patient said: *"Sounds like you got your hands full." "That must have been tough."* (Also implies that behavior is normal and gives symptom expectation.)

[1]Adapted from Carlat (2005).

18. Tactful use of language and wording, for example, being *"preoccupied,"* rather than "anxious;" or *"most of us hit a bump in life,"* rather than *"psychological problems are fairly common."*

19. Approach referral by building a case, for example, *"Mrs. Jones, based on the hearing testing, your reports of school difficulty, the score on the [PSC] rating form, and . . . I'm concerned about your child."* Perhaps add, *"How do you feel about it?"*

20. In suggesting referral, use indirect wording, for example, *"How about talking to an expert in that area?"* rather than, *"How about seeing a psychiatrist or psychologist,"* which are very emotionally weighted words.

21. Be sensitive to the understandable and widespread resistance to seeing a mental health professional. One can say, *"I can see you are not excited about that." "Can I ask what concerns you about that?" "That's a common reaction."*

22. Reassure. Patient/parent: *"You think (I'm)/she is crazy?"* Audiologist: *"Not at all. I just think there is something going on that seems worrisome, and I think we'd both like to get to the bottom of it."* Or, patient/parent: *"Shrinks try to get inside your head."* Audiologist: *"I think there are a lot of misconceptions about psychologists and psychiatrists. Actually, they are just good at helping people discover things, being supportive, and at finding ways to handle troublesome situations."*

Audiologists might be concerned that they will be perceived as prying or out of line. Yet, people probably can tell when a clinician is kind, sincere, and genuinely interested; as a result they won't be angry or offended. If a patient or parent becomes annoyed or hostile, it is not necessarily the audiologist's fault nor is it necessarily a bad outcome. It is not unusual for patients to direct their negative feelings to the person who is saying something they do not want to hear. Clinicians must not take it personally. Sometimes unpleasant news must be imparted, even though it is unwelcome. An audiologist must not be defensive or judgmental. One should validate those feelings. *"I can see how that would be upsetting."* Show that you are an ally: *"I might not like it either."* Explain your actions as arising from concern and that you regret making the person uncomfortable. None of this dialogue should be disingenuous; rather, it must be sincere, or it probably will come across as staged, which would make matters worse. In this clinician's 40 years of experience, patient and/or parent response has been overwhelmingly favorable.

Conclusion

In conclusion, if an audiologist has reasonable suspicion that a person is at risk for a psychosocial problem, remember the time-honored axiom: "If in doubt, refer." Referral to the person's primary care provider or to an appropriate professional then can be discussed with the patient or parent. Some might suppose that referral to a mental health professional may be harmful because of its unfortunate stigma. Yet, it is more likely that greater harm will be done by *not* referring. By missing the signs of risk or not acting on them, an audiologist might delay badly needed intervention and prolong distress. Conversely, by taking positive action and exploring for possible problems other than a hearing disorder, an audiologist may be the catalyst that gets a person the management he or she needs. Seen in this light, audiologists may find, as this one has, that dealing with matters of FEHL is not so much exasperating as deeply rewarding.

REFERENCES

Alberti, P. (1970). New tools for old tricks. *Annals of Otology, Rhinology and Laryngology*, *79*, 900–907.

American Academy of Otolaryngology Committee on Hearing and Equilibrium, and the American Council of Otolaryngology Committee on the Medical Aspects of Noise. (1979). Guide for the evaluation of hearing handicap. *Journal of the American Medical, Association*, 241(19), 2055–2059.

American Psychiatric Association. (2000). *Diagnostic and statistical manual of mental disorders* (Rev., 4th ed.). Washington, DC: Author.

American Speech-Language-Hearing Association. (2005). *Guidelines for manual pure-tone threshold audiometry*. Available from http://www.asha.org/policy.

Andaz, C., Heyworth, T., & Rowe, S. (1995). Nonorganic hearing loss in children—a 2 year study. *ORL Journal for Otorhinolaryngology and its Related Specialties*, *57*, 33–35.

Aplin, D. Y., & Rowson, V. J. (1986). Personality and functional hearing loss in children. *British Journal of Clinical Psychology*, *25*, 313–314.

Aplin, D. Y., & Rowson, V. J. (1990). Psychological characteristics of children with functional hearing loss. *British Journal of Audiology*, *24*, 77–87.

Austen, S., & Lynch, C. (2004). Non-organic hearing loss redefined: understanding, categorizing and managing non-organic behavior. *International Journal of Audiology*, *43*, 449–457.

Bagby, R. M., Wild, N., & Turner, A. (2003). Psychological assessment in adult mental health settings. In J. R. Graham & J. A. Nagliere (Eds.), I. B. Weiner (Editor-in-Chief), *Handbook of psychology, Volume 10, Assessment psychology* (pp. 213–234). Hoboken, NJ: John Wiley & Sons.

Balatsouras, D. G., Kaberos, A., Korres, S., Kandiloros, D., Ferekidis, E., & Economou, C. (2003). Dectection of pseudohypacusis: A prospective randomized study of the use of otoacoustic emissions. *Ear and Hearing*, *24*, 518–527.

Ban, J., & Jin, S. M. (2006). A clinical analysis of psychogenic sudden deafness. *Otolaryngology-Head and Neck Surgery*, *134*, 970–974.

Barelli, P. A., & Ruder, L. L. (1970). Medico-legal evaluation of hearing problems. *Eye, Ear, Nose and Throat Monthly*, *49*, 398–405.

Barr, B. (1960). Nonorganic hearing problems in school-children. Functional deafness. *Acta Oto-Laryngologica*, *52*, 337–346.

Barr, B. (1963). Psychogenic deafness in school-children. *International Audiology*, *2*, 125–128.

Beagley, H. A., & Knight, J. J. (1968) The evaluation of suspected non-organic hearing loss. *Journal of Laryngology and Otology*, *82*, 693–705.

Bengtzen, R., Woodward, M., Lynn, M. J., Newman, N. J., & Biousse, V. (2008). The "sunglasses sign" predicts nonorganic visual loss in neuro-ophthalmologic practice. *Neurology*, *70*, 218–221.

Berger, K. (1965). Pseudohypacusis in children. *Laryngoscope*, *75*, 447–457.

Berk, R. L. & Feldman, A. S. (1958). Functional hearing loss in children. *New England Journal of Medicine*, *259*, 214–216.

Berliner, L., & Elliott, D.M. (2002). Sexual abuse of children. In J. E. B. Myers, L. Berliner, J. Briere, C. T. Hendrix, C. Jenny, & T. A. Reid (Eds.), *The APSAC handbook on child maltreatmen*t (2nd ed., pp. 55–78). Thousand Oaks, CA: Sage.

Bowdler, D. A., & Rogers, J. (1989). The management of pseudohypacusis in school-age children. *Clinical Otolaryngology*, *14*, 211–215.

Brady, G. Y., Jr., & Wilson, R. G. (2004). The hearing care professional as an expert witness. *Hearing Review.* Available from http://www.hearingreview.com/issues/articles/2004-05_03.asp

Broad, R. D. (1980). Developmental and psychodynamic issues related to cases of childhood functional hearing loss. *Child Psychiatry and Human Development*, *11*, 49–58.

Brockman, S. J., & Hoversten, G. H. (1960). Pseudo neural hypacusis in children. *Laryngoscope*, *70*, 825–839.

Brooker, A.-S., Frank, J. W., & Tarasuk, V. S. (1997). Back pain claim rates and the business cycle. *Social Science Medicine*, *45*(3), 429–439.

Brooks D., & Geoghegan, P. M. (1993). Non-organic hearing loss in young persons: transient episode or indicator of deep-seated difficulty. *British Journal of Audiology*, *27*, 61.

Burk, M. H., & Wiley, T. L. (2004). Continuous versus pulsed tones in audiometry. *American Journal of Audiology*, *13*, 54–61.

Caceres, C. A., & Perry, L. W. (1967). *The innocent murmur: A problem in clinical practice*, Boston, MA: Little, Brown.

Campanelli, P. A. (1963). Simulated hearing losses in school children following identification audiometry. *Journal of Auditory Research*, *3*, 91–108.

Campbell, K. C. M. (1998). *Essential audiology for physicians.* San Diego, CA: Singular.

Campbell, K. C. M., Peck, J. E., & Lee, K. J. (2008). Audiology. In K. J. Lee (Ed.), *Essential otolaryngology head and neck surgery* (9th ed., pp. 24-69). New York, NY: McGraw-Hill Medical.

Campbell, R. J. (2004). *Psychiatric dictionary* (8th ed.). New York, NY: Oxford University Press.

Carhart, R. (1961). Tests for malingering. *Transactions of the American Academy of Ophthalmology and Otolaryngology, 65*, 437.

Carlat, J. D. (2005). *The psychiatric interview* (2nd ed.). Philadelphia, PA: Lippincott Williams & Wilkins.

Centers for Disease Control and Prevention. (2004). Methods of suicide among persons aged 10-19 years—United States, 1992-2001. *Morbidity and Mortality Weekly Report, 53*, 471-473.

Chaiklin, J. B. (1990). A descending LOT-Bekesy screening test for functional hearing loss. *Journal of Speech and Hearing Disorders, 55*, 67-74.

Chaiklin, J. B., & Ventry, I. M. (1965). Patient errors during spondee and pure-tone threshold measurement. *Journal of Auditory Research, 5*, 219-230.

Chawla, J. M., Handa, K. K., & Tripathi, B. M. (2007). Unilateral pseudohypacusis in children. *Indian Journal of Pediatrics, 74*, 312-313.

Cherry, R., & Ventry, I. M. (1976). The ascending-descending gap: A tool for identifying a suprathreshold response. *Journal of Auditory Research, 16*, 281-287.

Coles, R. (1993). NOHL: Definition and causes. In J. Ballantyne, M. C. Martin, & A. Martin (Eds.), *Deafness* (5th ed., pp. 216-218). London, UK: Whurr.

Coles, R. (2001). Non-organic hearing loss. In J. Graham & M. Martin (Eds.), *Ballantyne's deafness* (6th ed., pp. 239-245). London, UK: Whurr.

Cooper, C., Selwood, A., & Livingston, G. (2008). The prevalence of elder abuse and neglect: A systematic review. *Age and Ageing, 37*, 151-160.

Colman, A. M. (2001). *A dictionary of psychology.* Oxford, UK: Oxford University Press.

Corsini, R. J. (1999). *The dictionary of psychology.* Philadelphia, PA: Brunner/Mazel.

Czubak, M .F. (1923). The Stenger test for the detection of simulated unilateral total deafness. *Laryngoscope, 33*, 921-923.

Deaf Wannabee. (2008). Web site: http://groups.yahoo.com/group/DeafWannabee/

De Koker, E. (2004). *The clinical value of auditory steady state responses in the audiological assessment of pseudohypacusic workers with noise-induced hearing loss in the South African mining industry.* Doctoral thesis, University of Pretoria, South Africa. Available from: http://upetd.up.ac.za/thesis/available/etd-10152004-102003/.

DeRose, L. M., Wright, A. J., & Brooks-Gunn, J. (2006). Does puberty account for the gender differential in depression? In C. L. M. Keyes & S. H. Goodman (Eds.), *Women and depression: A handbook for the social, behavioral, and biomedical sciences* (pp. 89-128). Cambridge, UK: Cambridge University Press.

DiGiovanni, J. J., & Repka, J. N. (2007). Response method in audiometry. *American Journal of Audiology, 16*, 145-148.

Dixon, R. F., & Newby, H. A. (1959) Children with nonorganic hearing problems. *Archives of Otolaryngology, 70*, 619-623.

Dockum, G., & Robinson, D. (1975). Warble tone as an audiometric stimulus. *Journal of Speech and Hearing Disorders, 40*, 351-356.

Doebbeling, C. C. (2000). Epidemiology, risk factors, and prevention. In J. L. Levenson (Ed.), *Depression* (pp. 23-46). Philadelphia, PA: American College of Physicians.

Doerfler, L., & Stewart, K. (1946). Malingering and psychogenic deafness. *Journal of Speech Disorders, 11*, 181-186.

Domico, W. D. (1993). Legal issues in audiology. *Seminars in Hearing, 14*, 172-181.

Dorland's illustrated medical dictionary. (2003). 30th ed. Philadelphia, PA: Saunders.

Drake, A. F., Makielski, K., McDonald-Bell, C., & Atcheson, B. (1995). Two new otolaryngologic findings in child abuse. *Archives of Otolaryngology Head and Neck Surgery, 121*, 1417-1420.

Durmaz, A., Karahatay, S., Satar, B., Birkent, H., & Hidir, Y. (2009). Efficiency of Stenger test in confirming profound, unilateral pseudohypacusis. *Journal of Laryngology and Otology*, March 19, 2009. doi: 10.1017/S0022215109004769, Published online by Cambridge University Press, PMID: 19296863.

Durrant, J. D., Kesterson, R. K., & Kamerer, D. B. (1997). Evaluation of the nonorganic hearing loss suspect. *American Journal of Otology, 18*, 361-367.

Engelberg, M. W. (1970). *Audiological evaluation for exaggerated hearing level.* Springfield, IL: Charles C. Thomas.

English, K., & Clark, J.G. (2003). Counseling in audiology. The third ear. *Audiology Today, 15*, 29.

English, K., Mendel, L.L., Rojeski, T., & Hornak, J. (1999). Counseling in audiology, or learning to listen: Pre- and post-measures from an audiology counseling course. *American Journal of Audiology*, *8*, 34–39.

Erikson, M. F., & Egeland, B. (2002). Child neglect. In J. E. B. Myers, L. Berliner, J. Briere, C. T. Hendrix, C. Jenny, & T. A. Reid (Eds.), *The APSAC handbook on child maltreatment* (2nd ed., pp. 3–20). Thousand Oaks, CA: Sage.

Falconer, G.A. (1966). A "lipreading test" for nonorganic deafness. *Journal of Speech and Hearing Disorders*, *31*, 241–247.

Feder, H. A. (2000). Your role in the discovery process. In: *Succeeding as an expert* (pp. 117–123.) Glenwood Springs, CO: Tegeh Press.

Feldman, M. D., Eisendrath, S. J., & Tyerman, M. (2008). Psychiatric and behavioral correlates of factitious blindness. *Comprehensive Psychiatry*, *49*, 159–162.

Forke, C. M., Myers, R. K., Catallozzi, M., & Schwarz, D. F. (2008). Relationship violence among female and male college undergraduate students. *Archives of Pediatric and Adolescent Medicine*, *162*, 634–641.

Frank, T. (1976). Yes-no test for nonorganic hearing loss. *Archives of Otolaryngology*, *102*, 162–165.

Franklin, C., Johnson, K., Smith-Olinde, L., & Nicholson, N. (2009). The relationship of audiometric thresholds elicited with pulsed, warbled, and pulsed-warbled tones in adults with normal hearing. *Ear and Hearing*, *30*, 485–487.

Gale Group. (1998). *West's encyclopedia of American law* (2nd ed.). Detroit, MI: West Group.

Galloway, F. T., & Butler, R. A. (1956). Conditioned eyelid response to tone as an objective test of hearing. *Journal of Speech and Hearing Disorders*, *21*, 47–55.

Gaynor, E. B. (1974). Humming and nonorganic hearing loss. *Archives of Otolaryngology*, *100*, 199–200.

Gelfand, S A. (1993). Organic thresholds and functional components in experimentally simulated exaggerated hearing loss. *British Journal of Audiology*, *27*, 35–40.

Gelfand, S. A. (1998). *Hearing: An introduction to psychological and physiological acoustics* (3rd ed.). New York, NY: Marcel Dekker.

Gelfand, S. A., Schwander, T., & Silman, S. (1990). Acoustic reflex thresholds in normal and cochlear-impaired ears: Effects of no-response rates on 90th percentiles in a large sample. *Journal of Speech and Hearing Disorders*, *55*, 198–205.

Gelfand, S. A., & Silman, S. (1985). Functional hearing loss and its relationship to resolved hearing levels. *Ear and Hearing*, *6*, 151–158.

Gelfand, S. A., & Silman, S. (1993). Functional components and resolved thresholds in patients with unilateral nonorganic hearing loss. *British Journal of Audiology, 27,* 29–34.

Gleason, W. J. (1958). Psychological characteristics of the audiologically inconsistent patient. *Archives of Otolaryngology, 68,* 42–46.

Gold, S. R., Hunsacker, D. H., & Haseman, E. M. (1991). Pseudohypacusis in a military population. *Ear, Nose and Throat Journal, 70,* 710–712.

Goldstein, R. (1966). Pseudohypacusis. *Journal of Speech and Hearing Disorders, 31,* 341–352.

Goodhill, V. (Ed.). (1979). *Ear diseases deafness & dizziness.* Hagerstown, MD: Harper and Row.

Gordon, B. N., & Schroeder, C. S. (1995). *Sexuality: A developmental approach to problems.* New York, NY: Plenum Press.

Green, D. S. (1978). Pure tone air-conduction testing. In J. Katz (Ed.), *Handbook of clinical audiology* (2nd ed., pp. 98–109). Baltimore, MD: Williams & Wilkins.

Griffiths, P. G., & Eddyshaw, D. (2006). Medically unexplained visual loss in adult patients. *Eye, 18,* 859–860.

Guttman, J. (1928) A new method of determining unilateral deafness and malingering. *Laryngoscope, 38,* 686–687.

Hall, J. W., III. (2000). *Handbook of otoacoustic emissions.* San Diego, CA: Singular.

Hall J. W., III, & Swanepoel, D. (2009). *Objective assessment of hearing.* San Diego, CA: Plural.

Hallewell, J. D., Goetzinger, C. P., Allen, M. L., & Proud, G. O. (1966). The use of hypnosis in audiologic assessment. *Acta Oto-Laryngologica, 61,* 205–208.

Hamill, T., & Price, L. (2008). *The hearing sciences.* San Diego, CA: Singular.

Hamill, T. A., Karasick-Rush, S., & Segal, M. N. (1998). The Falconer "lipreading" test for nonorganic hearing loss. *Florida Journal of Communication disorders, 18,* 52–57.

Harris, D. A. (1958). A rapid and simple technique for the detection of nonorganic hearing loss. *Archives of Otolaryngology, 68,* 758–760.

Hart, S. N., Brassard, M. R., Binggeli, N. J., & Davidson, H. A. (2002). Psychological maltreatment. In J. E. B. Myers, L. Berliner, J. Briere, C. T. Hendrix, C. Jenny, & T. A. Reid (Eds.), *The APSAC handbook on child maltreatment* (2nd ed., pp. 79–104). Thousand Oaks, CA: Sage.

Harvey, M. A. (2008, July). How to refer patients successfully to mental health professionals. Available from: http://www.hearingreview.com/issues/articles/2008-07_02.asp.

Hasbrouck, J. M. (1989). Auditory perceptual problems in non-organic hearing disorder. *Laryngoscope*, *99*(Pt. 2), 855–860.

Hattler, K. W. (1968). The Type V Békésy pattern: The effects of loudness memory. *Journal of Speech and Hearing Research*, *11*, 567–575.

Hattler, K. W. (1970). Lengthened off-time: A self-recording screening device for nonorganicity. *Journal of Speech and Hearing Disorders*, *35*, 113–122.

Hattler, K. W., & Schuchman, G. I. (1971). Efficiency of the Stenger, Doerfler-Stewart and lengthened off-time Bekesy tests. *Acta Oto-Laryngologica*, *72*, 262–267.

Hiraumi, H., Tsuji, J., Kanemaru, S., Fujino, K., & Ito, J. (2007). Non-organic hearing loss. *Acta Oto-laryngologica*, *127*(Suppl. 557), 3–7.

Holder, G. E., Gale, R. P., Acheson, J. F., & Robson, A. G. (2009) Electrodiagnostic assessment in optic nerve disease. *Current Opinion in Neurology*, *22*, 3–10.

Holenweg, A., & Kompis, M. (2010). Non-organic hearing loss: New and confirmed findings. *European Archives of Otorhinolaryngology*, *267*, 1213–1219.

Honaker, J. A., Gilbert, J. M., & Staab, J. P. (2010). Chronic subjective dizziness versus conversion disorder: Discussion of clinical findings and rehabilitation. *American Journal of Audiology, 19*, 3–8.

Hood, W. H., Campbell, R. A., & Hutton, C. L. (1964). An evaluation of the Békésy ascending-descending gap. *Journal of Speech and Hearing Research*, *7*, 123–132.

Hopkinson, N. T. (1967). Comment on: "pseudohypacusis." *Journal of Speech and Hearing Disorders*, *32*, 293–294.

Hopkinson, N. T. (1973). Functional hearing loss. In J. Jerger (Ed.), *Modern developments in audiology* (2nd ed., pp. 175–210). New York, NY: Academic Press.

Hopkinson, N. T. (1978). Speech tests for pseudohypacusis. In J. Katz (Ed.), *Handbook of clinical audiology* (2nd ed., pp. 291–302). Baltimore, MD: Williams & Wilkins.

Hosoi, H., Tsuta, Y., Murata, K., & Levitt, H. (1999). Suggestion audiometry for non-organic hearing loss (pseudohypacusis) in children. *International Journal of Pediatric Otorhinolaryngology*, *47*, 11–21.

Hussey, J. M., Chang, J. J., & Kotch, J. B. (2006). Child maltreatment in the United States: Prevalence, risk factors, and adolescent health consequences. *Pediatrics*, *118*, 933–942.

Hutchinson, G.L. (2001). *Disorders of simulation: Malingering, factitious disorders, and compensation neurosis.* Madison, CT: Psychosocial Press.

Hyde, M. (1997). The N1 response and its applications. *Audiology & Neurotology, 2*, 281–307.

Hyde, M., Matsumoto, N., Alberti, P., & Li, Y. (1985). Auditory evoked potentials in audiometric assessment of compensation and medicolegal patients. *Annals of Otology, Rhinology and Laryngology, 95*, 514–519.

Jellinek, M. S., Murphy, J. M., Robinson, J., Feins, A., Lamb, S., & Fenton, T. (1988). Pediatric symptom checklist: Screening school-age children for psychosocial dysfunction. *Journal of Pediatrics, 112*, 201–209.

Jerger, J. (1960). Bekesy audiometry in analysis of auditory disorders. *Journal of Speech and Hearing Research, 3*, 275–287.

Jerger, J., Burney, L., Mauldin, L., & Crump, B. (1974). Predicting hearing loss from the acoustic reflex. *Journal of Speech and Hearing Disorders, 39*, 11–22.

Jerger, J., & Herer, G. (1961). Unexpected dividend in Békésy audiometry. *Journal of Speech and Hearing Disorders, 26*, 390–391.

Jerger, S., & Jerger, J. (1981). Functional hearing disorders. In *Auditory disorders: A manual for clinical evaluation* (pp. 51–58). Boston, MA: Little, Brown and Company.

Johnson, K. O., Work, W. P., & McCoy, G. (1956) Functional deafness. *Annals of Otology, Rhinology, and Laryngology, 65*, 154–170.

Kariya, S., Fukushima, K., Kawasaki, A., Kataoka, Y., & Nishizaki, K. (2008). Auditory steady-state responses to multiple simultaneous stimuli in children with functional or sensorineural hearing loss. *European Archives of Otorhinolaryngology, 265*, 769–773.

Kashani, J. H., Beck, N. C., Hoeper, E. W., Fallahi, C., Corcoran, C. M., McAllister, J. A., Rosenberg, T. K., & Reid, J. C. (1987). Psychiatric disorders in a community sample of adolescents. *American Journal of Psychiatry, 144*, 584–589.

Kesser, B. W., & Friedman, R. A. (2002). Functional disorders: Hearing loss. In A. M. Seiden, T. A. Tami, M. L. Pensak, R. T. Cotton, & J. L. Gluckman (Eds.), *Otolaryngology: The essentials* (pp. 33–43). New York, NY: Thieme.

Kinstler, D. P., Phelan, J. G., & Lavender, R. W. (1970). Efficiency of the Stenger tests in identification of functional hearing loss. *Journal of Auditory Research, 10*, 118–123.

Kinstler, D . P., Phelan, J. G., & Lavender, R. W. (1972). The Stenger and speech Stenger tests in functional hearing loss. *Audiology, 11*, 187–193.

Klotz, R. E., Koch, A. W., & Hackett, T. P. (1960), Psychogenic hearing loss in children: A preliminary report. *Annals of Otology, Rhinology and Laryngology, 69*, 199–205.

Kolko, D. J. (2002). Child physical abuse. In J. E. B. Myers, L. Berliner, J. Briere, C . T. Hendrix, C. Jenny, & T. A. Reid (Eds.), *The APSAC handbook on child maltreatment* (2nd ed., pp. 21-54). Thousand Oaks, CA: Sage.

Krahn, L. E., Li, H., & O'Connor, M. K. (2003). Patients who strive to be ill: Factitious disorder with physical symptoms. *American Journal of Psychiatry, 160*, 1163-1168.

Leavitt, J. A. (2006). Diagnosis and management of functional visual deficits. *Current Treatment Options in Neurology, 8*, 45-51.

Lehrer, N. D., Hirschenfang, S., Miller, M. H., & Radpour, S. (1964). Nonorganic hearing problems in adolescents. *Laryngoscope, 74*, 64-69.

Leshin, G. J. (1960). Childhood nonorganic hearing loss. *Journal of Speech and Hearing Disorders, 25*, 290-292.

Libow, J. A. (2003). Illness falsification in children: Pathways to prevention. In P. W. Halligan, C. Bass, & D. A. Oakley (Eds.), *Malingering and illness deception* (pp.147-155). Oxford. UK: Oxford University Press.

Lightfoot, G., & Kennedy, V. (2006). Cortical electric response audiometry hearing threshold estimation: Accuracy, speed, and the effects of stimulus presentation features. *Ear and Hearing, 27*, 443-456.

Lin, J., & Staecker, H. (2006). Nonorganic hearing loss. *Seminars in Neurology, 26*, 321-330.

Lumio, J. S., Jauhiainen, T, & Gelhar, K. (1969). Three cases of functional deafness in the same family. *Journal of Laryngology and Otology, 83*, 299-304.

Main, C. J. (2003). The nature of chronic pain: a clinical and legal challenge. In P. W. Halligan, C. Bass, & D. A. Oakley (Eds.), *Malingering and illness deception* (pp. 171-183). Oxford, UK: Oxford University Press.

Maisami, M., & Freeman, J. M. (1987). Conversion reactions in children as body language: A combined child psychiatry/neurology team approach to the management of functional neurologic disorders in children. *Pediatrics, 80*, 46-52.

Margolis, R. H. (1993). Detection of hearing impairment with the acoustic stapedial reflex. *Ear and Hearing, 14*, 3-10.

Maris, R. W., Berman, A. L., Silverman, M. M., & Nesbit, P. A. (2000). Age and the lifespan. In R. W. Maris, A. L. Berman, & M. M. Silverman (Eds.), *Comprehensive textbook of suicidology* (pp. 127-144). New York, NY: Guilford Press.

Martin, F. N. *Introduction to audiology* (6th ed.). Boston, MA: Allyn & Bacon.

Martin, F. N. (2009). Nonorganic hearing loss. In J. Katz, L. Medwetsky, R. Burkhard, & L. Hood, (Eds.), *Handbook of clinical audiology* (6th ed., pp. 699–711). Baltimore, MD: Lippincott Williams & Wilkins.

Martin, F. N., Champlin, C. A., & Marchbanks, T. (1998). A varying intensity story test for simulated hearing loss. *Journal of the American Academy of Audiology*, *7*, 39–44.

Martin, F. N., Champlin, C. A., & McCreery, T. M. (2001). Strategies used in feigning hearing loss. *Journal of the American Academy of Audiology*, *12*, 59–63.

Martin, F. N., & Clark, J. G. (2009). *Introduction to audiology* (10th ed.). Boston, MA: Allyn & Bacon.

Martin, F. N., & Monro, D. A. (1976) Authors' comments on effects of sophistication on Type V Bekesy patterns in simulated hearing loss. *Journal of Speech and Hearing Disorders*, *41*, 283.

Martin, F. N., & Shipp, D. B. (1982). The effects of sophistication on three threshold tests for subjects with simulated hearing loss. *Ear and Hearing*, *3*, 34–36.

Martin, J. S., Martin, F. N., & Champlin, C. A. (2000). The CON-SOT-LOT Test for nonorganic hearing loss. *Journal of the American Academy of Audiology*, *11*, 46–51.

Martin, N. A. (1946). Psychogenic deafness. *Annals of Otology, Rhinology, and Laryngology*, *55*, 81–89.

Maxwell, V. B., & Brooks, D. N. (1986). Hysterical deafness: An unusual presentation of stress in an air traffic control officer. *Aviation, Space, and Environmental Medicine*, *57*, 263–266.

McCann, J. T. (1998). *Malingering and deception in adolescents: Assessing credibility in clinical and forensic settings.* Washington, DC: American Psychological Association.

McCanna, D. L., & DeLapa, G. (1981). A clinical study of twenty-seven children exhibiting functional hearing loss. *Language, Speech, and Hearing Services in Schools*, *12*, 26–35.

Mehta, Z. (2003). Limitations of pure tone audiometry in detection of nonorganic hearing loss: A case study. *Contemporary Issues in Communication Sciences and Disorders*, *30*, 59–69.

Mehta, Z, & Martindale, R. (2005). Pediatric nonorganic hearing loss: Psychosocial issues and management. *Contemporary Issues in Communication Sciences and Disorders*, *32*, 11–21.

Mendel, L. L., Danhauer, J. L., & Singh, S. (1999). *Singular's illustrated dictionary of audiology.* San Diego, CA: Singular.

Mendelson, G. (1985). "Compensation neurosis." An invalid diagnosis. *Medical Journal of Australia*, *13*, 561–564.

Miller, A. L., Fox, M. S., & Chan, G. (1968). Pure tone assessments as an aid in detecting suspected non-organic hearing disorders in children. *Laryngoscope*, *78*, 2170–2176.

Miller, L. (2008). Crime victim trauma: Confounding symptoms and syndromes. In *Counseling crime victims: practical strategies for mental health professionals* (pp. 61–74). New York, NY: Springer.

Miller, L. (2008). Sick and tired: Mind-body syndromes in the workplace. In *From difficult to disturbed: Understanding and managing dysfunctional employees* (pp. 146–181), New York, NY: American Management Association.

Mineau, S. M., & Schlauch, R. S. (1997). Threshold measurements for patients with tinnitus: Pulsed or continuous tones. *American Journal of Audiology*, *6*, 52–56.

Monro, D. A., & Martin, F.N. (1977). Effects of sophistication on four tests for nonorganic hearing loss. *Journal of Speech and Hearing Disorders*, *42*, 528-534.

Monsell, E. M., & Herzon F. S. (1984). Functional hearing loss presenting as sudden hearing loss: A case report. *American Journal of Otology*, *5*, 407–410.

Morita, S., Suzuki, M., & Iizuka, K. (2010). Non-organic hearing loss in childhood. *International Journal of Pediatric Otorhinolaryngology*, *74*, 441–446.

Mosby's dictionary of medicine, nursing, and allied health. (7th ed.). (2004). St. Louis, MO: Mosby.

Musiek, F. E., Bornstein, S. P., & Rintelmann, W. F. (1995). Transient evoked otoacoustic emissions and pseudohypacusis. *Journal of the American Academy of Audiology*, *6*, 293–301.

Nagel, R. F. (1964). RRLJ—a new technique for the noncooperative patient. *Journal of Speech and Hearing Disorders*, *29*, 492–493.

National Center for Injury Prevention and Control. (2006). *Sexual violence: Fact sheet.* Available from: http://www.cdc.gov/ncipc/factsheets.

National Institute of Mental Health. (2008). *The numbers count: Mental disorders in America. (2008).*Washington, DC: National Institutes of Health. Available from: http://www.minh.nih.gov.

National Spasmodic Torticollis Association. (2007, February). Available from: http://www.torticollis.org.

Nemzer, E. D. (1996). Somatoform disorders. In M. Lewis (Ed.), *Child and adolescent psychiatry: A comprehensive textbook* (2nd ed., pp. 693–702). Baltimore, MD: Williams & Wilkins.

Nilo, E. R., & Saunders, W. H. (1976). Functional hearing loss. *Laryngoscope*, *86*, 501–505.

Nober, E. H. (1970). Cutile air and bone conduction thresholds of the deaf. *Exceptional Children, 36*, 571–579.

Noble, W. (1987). The conceptual problem of "functional hearing loss." *British Journal of Audiology, 21*, 1–3.

Noble, W. G. (1978). *Assessment of impaired hearing: A critique and a new method.* New York, NY: Academic Press.

Oishi, N., Kanzaki, S., Kataoka, C., Tazoe, M., Takei, Y., Nagai, K., Kohno, N., & Ogawa K. (2009). Acute-onset unilateral psychogenic hearing loss in adults: Report of six cases and diagnostic pitfalls. *Otology, Rhinology, and Laryngology, 71*, 279–283.

Olsen, W .O. (1991). Special auditory tests: A historical perspective. In J. T. Jacobson & J. L. Northern (Eds.), *Diagnostic audiology* (pp. 19–51). Austin, TX: Pro-Ed.

Orchik, D. J, & Rintelmann, W. F. (1978). Comparison of pure-tone, warbled-tone and narrow-band noise thresholds of young normal-hearing children. *Journal of the American Audiological Society, 3*, 214–220.

Peck, J. E. (2002, April). *Pseudohypacusis: Psychosocial aspects.* Instructional course presented at the annual convention of the American Academy of Audiology, Philadelphia, PA.

Peck, J. E., & Ross, M. (1970). The ascending and descending methods for administering the pure tone Stenger test. *Journal of Auditory Research, 5*, 218–220.

Pracy, J. P., Walsh, R. M., Mepham, G. A., & Bowdler, D. A. (1996). Childhood pseudohypacusis. *International Journal of Pediatric Otorhinolaryngology, 37*,143–149.

Priebe, G., & Svedin, C. G. (2008). Child sexual abuse is largely hidden from the adult society. An epidemiological study of adolescents' disclosures. *Child Abuse and Neglect, 32*, 1095–1108.

Psarommatis, I., Kontorinis, G., Kontrogiannis, A., Douniadakis, D., & Tsakanikos, M. (2009). Pseudohypacusis: The most frequent etiology of sudden hearing loss in children. *European Archives of Oto-Rhino-Laryngology, 266*, 1857–1861.

Qiu, W. W., Stucker, F. J., Yin, S. S., & Welsh, L. W. (1998). Current evaluation of pseudohypacusis: strategies and classification. *Annals of Otology, Rhinology, and Laryngology, 107*, 638–647.

Rabinoff, M. A., & Holmes, S. P. (1996). *The forensic expert's guide to litigation: The anatomy of a lawsuit.* Danvers, MA: LRP Publications.

Radkowski, D, Cleveland, S., & Friedman, E. M. (1998). Child pseudohypacusis in patients with high risk for actual hearing loss. *Laryngoscope, 108*, 1534–1538.

Raine, A. (2003). Malingering and criminal behaviour as psychopathology. In P. W. Halligan, C. Bass, & D. A. Oakley (Eds.), *Malingering and illness deception* (pp. 93-106). Oxford, UK: Oxford University Press.

Read, J., McGregor, K., Coggan, C., & Thomas, D. R. (2006). Mental health services and sexual abuse: The need for staff training. *Journal of Trauma and Dissociation*, 7, 33-50.

Rickards, F. W., deVidi, S., & McMahon, D. S. (1996). Audiologic indicators of exaggerated hearing loss in noise induced hearing loss claims. *Australian Journal of Audiology, 18*, 89-97.

Riedner E. D., & Efros, P. L. (1995). Nonorganic hearing loss and child abuse: Beyond the sound booth. *British Journal of Audiology, 29*, 195-197.

Rintelmann, W., & Harford, E. R. (1963). The detection and assessment of pseudohypacusis among school-age children. *Journal of Speech and Hearing Disorders, 28*, 141-152.

Rintelmann, W. F., & Harford, E. R. (1967). Type V Békésy pattern: Interpretation and clinical utility. *Journal of Speech and Hearing Research, 10*, 733-746.

Rintelmann, W. F., & Schwan S. A. (1991). Pseudohypacusis. In W. F. Rintelmann (Ed.), *Hearing assessment* (2nd ed., pp. 603-652). Boston, MA: Allyn & Bacon.

Rintelmann, W. F., & Schwan, S. A. (1999). Pseudohypacusis. In F. E. Musiek & W. F. Rintelmann (Eds.) *Contemporary perspectives in hearing assessment* (pp. 415-435). Boston, MA: Allyn & Bacon.

Robinette, M. S., & Gaeth, J. H. (1972). Diplacusis and the Stenger test. *Journal of Auditory Research, 12*, 91-100.

Roeser, R. J., Buckley, K. A, & Stickney, G. S. (2000). Pure tone tests. In R. J. Roeser, M. Valente, & H. Hosford-Dunn (Eds.), *Audiology diagnosis* (pp. 227-251). New York, NY: Thieme.

Rogers, R., & Neumann, C. S. (2003). Conceptual issues and explanatory models of malingering. In P. W. Halligan, C. Bass, & D. A. Oakley (Eds.), *Malingering and illness deception* (pp. 71-82). Oxford, UK: Oxford University Press.

Ross, M. (1964). The variable intensity pulse count method (VIPCM) for the detection and measurement of the pure tone threshold of children with functional hearing losses. *Journal of Speech and Hearing Disorders, 29*, 477-482.

Ruhm, H. B., & Cooper, W. A., Jr. (1962). Low sensation level effects of pure-tone delayed auditory feedback. *Journal of Speech and Hearing Research, 5*, 185-193.

Ruhm, H. B., & Cooper, W. A., Jr. (1964). Delayed feedback audiometry. *Journal of Speech and Hearing Disorders*, *29*, 448–455.

Sacks, M. E. (1995). An overview of the law: *A guide for testifying and consulting experts* (pp. 11–22). Danvers, MA: LRP Publications.

Sadock, B. J., & Sadock, V. A. (2008). Somatoform disorders. In *Kaplan & Sadock's concise textbook of clinical psychiatry* (3rd ed., pp. 273–286). Philadelphia, PA: Lippincott Williams & Wilkins.

Sakashita, T., Shibata, T., Yamane, H., & Hashimoto, C. (2004). Usefulness of otoacoustic emissions in diagnosis of pseudohypacusis with organic hearing loss; A report of two cases. *Practica Otologica (Kyoto)*, *97*, 105–112.

Sanders, J. W., & Lazenby, B. B. (1983). Auditory brain stem response measurement in the assessment of pseudohypacusis. *American Journal of Otology*, *4*, 292–299.

Saravanappa, N., Mepham, G. A., & Bowdler, D. A. (2005). Diagnostic tools in pseudohypacusis in children. *International Journal of Pediatric Otorhinolaryngology*, *69*, 1235–1238.

Saunders, G. H., Field, D. L., & Haggard, M. P. (1992). A clinical test battery for obscure auditory dysfunction (OAD): Development, selection and use of tests. *British Journal of Audiology*, *26*, 33–42.

Saunders, G. H., & Forsline, A. (2006). The performance-perceptual test (PPT) and its relationship to aided reported handicap and hearing aid satisfaction. *Ear and Hearing*, *27*, 229–242.

Saunders, G. H., Forsline, A., & Fausti, S. A. (2004). The performance-perceptual test and its relationship to unaided reported handicap. *Ear and Hearing 25*, 117–126.

Saunders, G. H., & Haggard, M. P. (1989). The clinical assessment of obscure auditory dysfunction—1. Auditory and psychological factors. *Ear and Hearing 10*, 200–208.

Saunders, G. H., & Haggard, M. P. (1992). The assessment of "Obscure Auditory Dysfunction" (OAD) 2. Case control analysis of determining factors. *Ear and Hearing*, *13*, 241–254.

Saunders, G. H., & Haggard, M. P. (1993). The influence of personality-related factors upon consultation for two different "marginal" organic pathologies with and without reports of auditory symptomatology. *Ear and Hearing*, *14*, 242–248.

Schlauch, R. S., Arnce, K. D., Olson, L. M., Sanchez, S., & Doyle, T. N. (1996). Identification of pseudohypacusis using speech recognition thresholds. *Ear and Hearing*, *17*, 229–236.

Schneider, R. K., & Levenson, J. L. (2008). *Psychiatric essentials for primary care.* Philadelphia, PA: American College of Physicians.

Shahrokh, N. C., & Hales, R. E. (Eds.). (2003). *American psychiatric glossary* (8th ed.). Washington, DC: American Psychiatric Publishing.

Sharpe, M. (2003). Distinguishing malingering from psychiatric disorders. In P. W. Halligan, C. Bass, & D. A. Oakley (Eds.), *Malingering and illness deception* (pp. 156-170). Oxford, UK: Oxford University Press.

Siegel, J. G., & Shim, J. K. (2005). *Dictionary of accounting terms* (4th ed.). Hauppauge, NY: Barron's Educational Series.

Silver, F. W. (1996). Management of conversion disorder. *American Journal of Physical Medicine and Rehabilitation*, *75*, 134-140.

Silverman, J. G., Raj, A., Mucci, L. A., & Hathaway, J. E. (2001, August 1). Dating violence against adolescent girls and associated substance use, unhealthy weight control, sexual risk behavior, pregnancy, and suicidality. *Journal of the American Medical Association*, *286*, 572-579.

Snyder, J. M. (1973). Interaural attenuation characteristics in audiometry. *Laryngoscope*, *83*, 1847-1855.

Snyder, J. M. (2001). Audiological evaluation for exaggerated hearing loss. In R. A. Dobie (Ed.), *Medical-legal evaluation of hearing loss* (2nd ed., pp. 49-88). San Diego, CA: Singular Thomson Learning.

Sood, A. A., & Sood, R. K. (2000). Depression in children and adolescents. In J. L. Levenson (Ed.), *Depression* (pp. 225-250). Philadelphia, PA: American College of Physicians.

Spraggs, P. D. R., Burton, M. J., & Graham, J. M. (1994). Nonorganic hearing loss in cochlear implant candidates. *American Journal of Otology*, *15*, 652-657.

Stach, B. A. (2003). *Comprehensive dictionary of audiology: Illustrated* (2nd ed.). Clifton Park, NY: Delmar Learning.

Stapells, D. R., & Oates, P. (1997). Estimation of the pure-tone audiogram by the brainstem response: A review. *Audiology and Neurotology*, *2*, 257-280.

Stephens, D., Zhao, F., & Kennedy, V. (2003). Is there an association between noise exposure and King Kopetzky syndrome? *Noise Health*, *5*, 55-62. Retrieved April 20, 2008. Available from: http://www.noiseandhealth.org/text.asp?2003/5/20/55/31688.

Sutherland, A. J., & Rodin, G. M. (1990). Factitious disorders in a general hospital setting: Clinical features and a review of the literature. *Psychosomatics*, *31*, 392-399.

Taich, A., Crowe, S., Kosmorsky, G. S., & Traboulsi, E. I. (2004). Prevalence of psychosocial disturbances in children with nonorganic visual loss. *Journal of the American Association for Pediatric Ophthalmology and Strabismus*, *8*, 457-461.

Taylor, G. J. (1949). An experimental study of tests of the detection of auditory malingering. *Journal of Speech and Hearing Disorders, 14*, 119–130.

Thomas, C. S. (2002). Psychological consequences of traumatic injury. [Editorial]. *British Journal of Psychiatry, 180*, 392–393.

Thompson, G., & Denman, M. (1970). The occlusion effect in unilateral functional hearing loss. *Journal of Speech and Hearing Research, 13*, 37–40.

Tilkian, A. G., & Conover, M. B. (2001). *Understanding heart sounds and murmurs with an introduction to lung sounds* (4th ed.). Philadelphia, PA: W. B. Saunders.

Trier, T. R., & Levy, R. (1965). Social and psychological characteristics of veterans with functional hearing loss. *Journal of Auditory Research, 5*, 241–256.

U.S. Department of Commerce. (2004). *Statistical abstract of the United States: 2004–2005* (124th ed.). Washington, DC: Author.

U.S. National Center for Health Statistics, Centers for Disease Control and Prevention. (2008). *National suicide statistics at a glance.* Available from: http://www.cdc.gov/nchs/.

Veniar, F. A., & Salston, R. S. (1983). An approach to the treatment of pseudohypacusis in children. *American Journal of Diseases in Children, 137*, 34–36.

Ventry, I. M. (1968). A case for psychogenic hearing loss. *Journal of Speech and Hearing Disorders, 33*, 89–92.

Ventry, I. M. (1976a). Comment on article by Martin and Monro. *Journal of Speech and Hearing Disorders, 41*, 282.

Ventry, I. M. (1976b). Pure tone-spondee threshold relationships in functional hearing loss: A hypothesis. *Journal of Speech and Hearing Disorders, 41*, 16–22.

Ventry, I. M., & Chaiklin, J. B. (1962). Functional hearing loss: A problem in terminology. *Asha, 4*, 251–254.

Ventry, I. M., & Chaiklin, J. B. (1965a). Efficiency of audiometric measures used to identify functional hearing loss. *Journal of Auditory Research, 5*, 196–211.

Ventry, I. M., & Chaiklin, J. B. (1965b). Evaluation of pure-tone audiogram configurations used in identifying adults with functional hearing loss. *Journal of Auditory Research, 5*, 212–218.

Ventry, I. M., & Chaiklin, J. B. (1965c). Introduction and research plan. *Journal of Auditory Research, 5*, 179–190.

Ventry, I. M., & Chaiklin, J.B. (1965d). Multidiscipline study of functional hearing loss. *Journal of Auditory Research*, *5*, 179–272.

Villegas, R. B., & Ilsen, P. F. (2008). Functional vision loss: A diagnosis of exclusion. *Optometry*, *79*, 123.

Wang, Y-P, Wang, M-C., Lin, H-C., & Lee, K-S. (2006). Conversion deafness presenting as sudden hearing loss. *Journal of the Chinese Medical Association*, *69*, 289–293.

Waslick, B. D., Kandel, R., & Kakouros, A. (2002). Depression in children and adolescents: An overview. In D. Shaffer, & B. D. Waslick (Eds.), *The many faces of depression in children and adolescents* (pp. 1–36). Washington, DC: American Psychiatric Publishing.

Weiss, B. G. (1971). Predicating organic hearing levels: The Falconer lipreading test for nonorganic deafness. *Journal of Auditory Research*, *11*, 223–226.

Wilbur, L. A. (1994). Calibration in clinical audiology. In J. Katz (Ed.), *Handbook of clinical audiology* (4th ed., pp. 73–94). Baltimore, MD: Williams & Wilkins.

Wolf, M., Birger, M., Ben-Shoshan, J., & Kronenberg, J. (1993). Conversion deafness. *Annals of Otology, Rhinology and Laryngology*, *102*, 349–352.

Woodford, C. M., Harris, G., Marquette, M. L., Perry, L., & Barnhart, M. (1997). A screening test for pseudohypacusis. *Hearing Review*, *11*, 23–24, 26.

World Health Organization. (2001). *International statistical classification of diseases and related health problems-10th Revision (ICD-10).* Geneva, Switzerland: Author.

Yoshida, M., Noguchi, A., & Uemura, A. (1989). Functional hearing loss in children. *International Journal of Pediatric Otorhinolaryngology*, *17*, 287–295.

INDEX

B

C

D

J

L

M

N

R

S

T

U

V

W